TOP PRAISE
FOR *TOP SHAPE* MASTER
JOYCE L. VEDRAL!

"JUST LOOK WHAT YOU CAN DO IN MINUTES A DAY. THE ROUTINE WILL GET YOUR ENTIRE BODY HARD, TIGHT, AND RIPPED."
> —ROBERT KENNEDY,
> editor of *Musclemag International*
> and author of *Rock Hard*

"*TOP SHAPE* IS THE ULTIMATE TOTAL-BODY FITNESS MANUAL."
> —LUD SHUSTERICH,
> world powerlifting record holder, and member of
> All Time Greats Bodybuilding Hall of Fame

"THE BEST 30–40 MINUTES YOU'LL EVER INVEST. With *TOP SHAPE*, in 3–4 weekly sessions, you will not only reverse the aging process, but have a better body than you did in your twenties. I recommend this book to all my patients."
> —DR. JUDE BARBERA, M.D.,
> urologist and professor of surgery,
> Downstate Medical Center, Brooklyn, New York

"AS A COSMETIC SURGEON, I STRONGLY ENDORSE THE TECHNIQUES OF WORKING OUT PRESENTED IN *TOP SHAPE*, not only as a way of looking great, but of maintaining and developing the overall body musculature that improves posture, overall strength, and energy level."
> —DR. GERALD ACKER, M.D., P.C.,
> director of cosmetic surgery,
> Long Beach Memorial Hospital, Long Beach, New York

"AS A MEMBER OF THE PRESIDENT'S COUNCIL ON PHYSICAL FITNESS AND A DOCTOR OF CHIROPRACTIC, I GIVE *TOP SHAPE* THE TOP GRADE!"
> —JACK BARNATHAN,
> doctor of chiropractic,
> chairman, Nassau County Council of Physical Fitness

"I RECOMMEND *TOP SHAPE* TO ALL MY CLIENTS."
> —GUS STEFANIDIS,
> Mr. Greece

TOP SHAPE

12 Weeks to Your Ideal Physique

Joyce L. Vedral., Ph.D.

WARNER BOOKS

A Time Warner Company

A NOTE FROM THE PUBLISHER

The information herein is not intended to replace the services of trained health care professionals. You are advised to consult with your health care professional with regard to matters relating to your health, and in particular regarding matters which may require diagnosis or medical attention.

Copyright © 1995 by Joyce L. Vedral, Ph.D.
All rights reserved.

Warner Books, Inc., 1271 Avenue of the Americas, New York, NY 10020

W A Time Warner Company

Printed in the United States of America
First Printing: March 1995
10 9 8 7 6 5 4 3

Library of Congress Cataloging-in-Publication Data

Vedral, Joyce L.
    Top shape : 12 weeks to your ideal physique / Joyce L.
Vedral.
        p.   cm.
    Includes bibliographical references and index.
    ISBN 0-446-39533-1
    1. Physical fitness for men.   2. Exercise for men.   I. Title.
GV482.5.V43   1995
613.7′0449—dc20   94-25011
                                                    CIP

Cover design by Diane Luger
Cover, introduction, and free weight exercise photos by Don Banks, New York
Machine workout photos by Chuck Rausin, California
Hair and makeup by Jody Pollutro
Cover, introduction, and free weight model: Franklin Rice
Machine workout model: Michael Lawton
Book design by Giorgetta Bell McRee

To the "before" and "after" men in this book,
and to the hundreds of thousands of men who are now in the "before" state,
but will soon, with a little dedication, become an "after."
I congratulate you ahead of time!

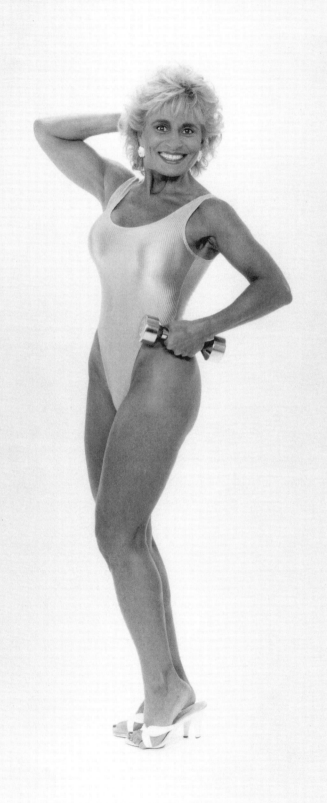

Acknowledgments

To Joann Davis, for your vision for this project.

To Grace Sullivan, for your cheerful, good-natured assistance.

To Diane Luger and Jackie Merri Meyer, for your creative cover art.

To Larry Kirshbaum, Nanscy Neiman, and Ellen Herrick, for your continual enthusiasm and support.

To Robin Laimo, director of the Garden City Saks Fifth Avenue Club, for helping me to dress for success!

To Edna Farley, for your talented handling of the publicity.

To Tom Terwilliger, national fitness champion, of Maximum Fitness, Boulder, Colorado, for being there for me from the very start.

To Carl Lewis, for offering thoughtful advice as to what men are really looking for in a workout.

To the hundreds of men who have written to me asking me to write such a book—thank you for your suggestions. I have shaped this book to your requests.

To the hundreds of women who have asked me to write a book for the men in their lives.

To the "before" and "after" men in this book, for being an inspiration to all men, and to the many "before" and "after" men who sent me their photographs but who do not appear in this book. To each of you, congratulations.

To Joe and Betty Weider, for inventing and promoting the training principles used in this book, and by the champions, and for your wonderful magazines, *Muscle and Fitness*, *Men's Fitness, Flex*, and *Shape*.

To Ken's Fitness Centre in Farmingdale, Long Island, for providing the perfect environment for working out—for both men and women.

To Family Fitness Center in Las Vegas, Nevada, for providing a fine workout environment for all!

To Canyon Ranch, for providing a place where men and women can go for a refreshing health and fitness retreat, and to Cathrine Brumley for providing a fine fitness program at Canyon Ranch in the Berkshires.

To Joan Mikus, administrator of the Pritikin Longevity Center, in Miami Beach, and to Dr. Robert Bauer and Dr. David Lehr, medical co-directors, for providing a place where health and fitness can be achieved and maintained.

To Don Banks, for your creative photography.

To Jody Pollutro for your wonderful work in hair and makeup.

To family and friends, for your continual love and support.

Contents

TOP
SHAPE

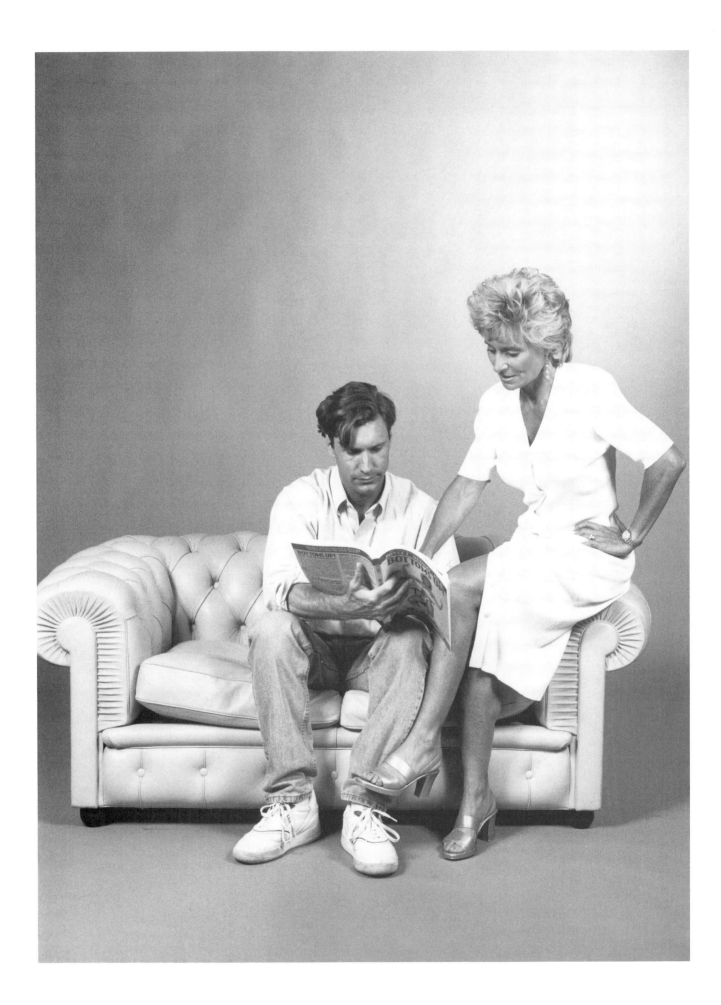

1

Top Shape

Most men don't want to look like bodybuilders, but they would like to be in top shape. In other words, they would like to look fit and be at least moderately muscular, and they would like to have some definition. And those men who are past thirty, and may now be in their forties, fifties, sixties, or older, would love to regain the body of their youth.

Well, regardless of your age, I have good news for you. Not only can you get into top, moderately muscular, well-defined shape, but you can have the best body you've ever had in your life—by working out with weights only three days a week for forty power-packed minutes, or four days a week for thirty minutes—a total of only two hours a week no matter which plan you choose!

Perhaps the best part of it all is, it won't take you forever to achieve your top shape. You can do it in twelve to twenty-four weeks, and if you follow the program exactly, I guarantee the results. Take a look at the before-and-after men in Chapter 2. They are the proof that what I'm telling you is true.

The workout is done at home with a minimum of equipment—only three sets of dumbbells and a bench. That's it! And for those of you who prefer going to a fitness center, or who like to work out on home-gym machines, a special chapter shows you how to use such equipment in order to achieve the maximum results.

WHAT I MEAN BY TOP SHAPE

The title of this book has a double meaning. The first meaning has already been explained—if you follow the workout contained in this book, you will achieve your top shape or dream shape. The second meaning of the title comes from the fact that the basic workout does not require you to exercise your legs—but rather your "top," or upper body: chest, shoulders, arms (biceps and triceps), back, and abdominals. A complete leg workout (front and back thighs and calves) is provided, but is optional. Why so?

From the hundreds of men I've interviewed, I learned that most men are not as concerned with the shape and size of their legs as they are with the shape and size of their upper bodies. For one thing, when a man looks at himself in the mirror each morning as he shaves, it is not his legs that he sees, but his upper body. For another, when a man gets dressed, whether in a suit, in pants and a fitted shirt, or in jeans and a T-shirt, it is the shape of his upper body, and not the shape of the muscles of his legs, that is clearly outlined.

In addition, some men tell me that although they realize that their legs could use some work, they don't really care that their legs are not as muscular as their upper bodies because their legs look "good enough," and also, if they don't wear shorts or a bathing suit very often, the shape of their legs is for the most part hidden.

Other men tell me that they are already doing some work for their legs—they are either jogging, running, riding an exercise bike, or using a stair-stepper. Such men realize that although these aerobic activities can never put significant muscle on their legs, at least their legs are strengthened by these activities.

The men are absolutely right. All of the above is true. Unless you are concerned with total-body symmetry, or unless your legs are particularly weak, there is no reason for you to force yourself to do the leg workout. Of course, being the fitness idealist and dreamer that I am, I hope that at some point, after you get your upper body into top shape, you say to yourself, "I think I'll get my legs in top shape too." But you don't have to do it. The choice is yours. The leg workout in this book is optional.

WHAT YOU WILL GET FROM THIS PROGRAM

- A reshaped body in twelve to twenty-four weeks of working out two hours a week
- Symmetrical muscularity and definition
- Increased metabolism due to muscle gain, so you can eat more without getting fat
- A low-fat, never-go-hungry eating plan
- Stronger bones and a healthier heart and lungs

- Improved posture, walk, and stance
- Reversal of the aging process on muscle and bone
- Lowered blood-pressure and cholesterol levels
- Freedom from measuring devices such as the scale, the fat-caliper, and the tape measure: the mirror and your clothing will be your new measurement
- Increased strength and improved performance in your sport
- Increased mental energy and a more positive outlook on life

WHY WHAT YOU HAVE BEEN DOING HAS NOT WORKED

Many of you have been going to fitness centers for years, and have been spending up to two hours per workout session, six hours a week, and still you are not in shape. Why not? Simply put, it's not the time you put in, but the method that counts. In other words, you have to do the right thing to get the right results.

For example, you can get some wood, a hammer, and some nails, and swing a hammer all day, banging nails into wood at random, but you won't get anything for your effort except a sore arm unless you are following a good plan. If you have such a plan and swing the hammer, pounding the nails into specific boards for a specific purpose, you can accomplish the spectacular!

Chances are, you've been doing various cardiovascular exercises, participating in several sports, engaging in circuit-training workouts, or random weight training, and nothing has happened, at least not the right things.

That was the case with the before-and-after men you will meet in Chapter 2. When I first met one of them, he bragged, "I work out for over an hour a day." Yet his body exhibited no outward sign of a bodyshaping workout. When I questioned him about his routine, it turned out that not only was he working out randomly (a chest exercise, a biceps exercise, a back exercise, and then another chest exercise), but he didn't know the purpose of some of the exercises. For example, he thought that the lat pulldown, a back exercise, was for his side abdominals, his "love handles." He had been working in this way for over a year, with, of course, no visible change in his body. He is now a proud "after" in Chapter 2.

WHY DOES THIS PROGRAM WORK?

This program is based upon the scientifically proven principles discovered by Joe Weider, publisher of *Muscle and Fitness* magazine, and used by all champion bodybuilders for the past fifty years. They are: muscle isolation, the pyramid system, and the forty-eight-hour recovery principle (or the split routine). They are simple to understand and easy to apply. Let us consider each one individually.

The **muscle isolation** principle requires that you work each muscle in isolation from all other muscles. In other words, you do a minimum amount of exercises for a given body part before moving on to the next body part. The point is, it is not wise to skip around at random, or to do a circuit-training type of routine where you exercise each body part once or twice, and then skip to the next body part, and perhaps later return to the original body part. Such a method does not supply enough "isolation" to force the working muscle to grow and change. In the Top Shape Workout, you will be doing a minimum of three to five exercises per body part, and you will do them without skipping around to other body parts.

The **pyramid system** requires that you add some weight to each set of a given exercise, as you decrease the number of repetitions. This system reduces boredom, but more important, it guarantees that you will get the most out of your working muscle with the least amount of strain. The psychology is, you are asked to lift a slightly heavier weight in the next set, but you are required to do fewer repetitions, so you say to yourself, "I can handle this." The method allows your muscles to be coaxed into working up to their fullest capacity. The pyramid system also provides a natural warm-up stretch, because your first set is light. In other words, you save time by eliminating a separate, elaborate warm-up stretching routine.

The **forty-eight-hour recovery principle**. This principle requires that you leave forty-eight hours of rest time for every exercised muscle (except abdominals, which can be exercised every day because these muscles are very small), in order to prevent muscle attrition (the wearing away of muscle) due to overtraining. In other words, you must leave a day's rest before doing another weight-training workout for any given muscle.

Since bodybuilders like to work out every day, and are required to lift very heavy weights, and do double the number of exercises required in this routine, and since they all work their legs in addition to their upper bodies, thus adding to the number of exercises they must do, they cannot possibly exercise all the muscles on one day and then take the next day off from working out with weights. Instead, they split the body into halves, working one half of the muscles on workout day one, and the other half of the body on workout day two. In this way they get to work all of their muscles without violating the forty-eight-hour rest principle. Their method is called the **split routine**, and it will be discussed next.

Since you are not going to be using extremely heavy weights or doing as many exercises as bodybuilders, and if you have not chosen to do the optional leg workout, you can perform your entire workout in one day and have the luxury of taking the next day off. Your advantage is, you can work out just three days a week, and your entire workout will take only forty minutes. All you have to do is leave one day between each workout. In other words, you can work out on Monday, Wednesday, and Friday, or Sunday, Tuesday, Thursday—or some such combination. (You can either rest on your "off" days, or you can do optional aerobic activities or sports. See pp. 66–68 for more about this.)

The Split Routine Option

As mentioned above, the split routine requires that you exercise approximately one half of the body on workout day one, and the other half of the body on workout day two. Although you are not a bodybuilder, and do not lift heavy weights, you may choose to do the split routine because you enjoy a shorter workout and feel that you can give more relaxed concentration to each muscle group by doing half of your body on workout day one, and the other half of your body on workout day two.

Another reason for choosing the split routine is to make the workout shorter if you have chosen to do the optional Ironman and/or Superman routines, which each add ten minutes or more to your workout time. (See p. 58 for an explanation of these routines.)

When the Split Routine Is Not an Option

If you have chosen to do the leg workout, you must use the split routine. To try to exercise eight body parts in one workout session would force you to cheat the last few body parts out of a good workout. By the end of the workout, you would simply be too tired to concentrate enough to gain the full benefit of the exercises. So if you've chosen to do the optional leg workout, the split routine is not an option. You must use it!

GO TO THE EXPERT

Why should you believe that any of the above principles are true—that working this way will actually help to reshape your body? The answer is clear. If you had a foot problem, you probably would not go to a doctor who specializes in general medicine, you would go to a doctor who specializes in feet—a podiatrist. If you had a heart problem, again, you would not go to a general practitioner, but you would instead seek out a cardiologist.

The same logic applies if you are seeking to attain your ideal physique. Why go to general fitness practitioners? Does it not make more sense to go to someone who is a proven expert in bodyshaping? I am that expert. Let me explain.

I have transformed my own body by using these principles. I have trained with and interviewed champion bodybuilders for years. I have written numerous training articles for magazines such as *Muscle and Fitness, Shape, Men's Fitness,* and *Musclemag,* and I've written several best-selling books on the subject, and these books—*Gut Busters, The Fat-Burning Workout, Bottoms Up!* (see bibliography for others)—have helped thousands of men and women transform their bodies into their ideal forms—and yet none of these men and women look like bodybuilders. Why not? Because my programs don't ask you to take the bodybuilding principles to the extreme. You are not asked to put in as many hours as do bodybuilders, and you are not asked to lift extremely heavy weights. But you are (and this point cannot possibly be exaggerated) asked to follow the exact same training principles as those used by champion bodybuilders. It is these principles that are the key to reshaping the body. They are the guaranteed way to get the results.

Why am I so sure? Bodybuilders have taken years to perfect the science of bodyshaping. For example, if a bodybuilder goes into a contest and his chest is too small in proportion to the rest of his body, he knows exactly how to go back to the weights and create larger chest muscles. If he loses a contest because his shoulders are not well developed, he knows exactly how to go to the weights and create the perfectly shaped shoulder, and so on. Nothing about his work is hit-and-miss, because he is using a science that has been developed over the past fifty years—a science that inevitably works if applied as directed.

WHY DO OTHER WORKOUTS FAIL TO RESHAPE THE BODY?

Okay. Now that you know why this program does work to reshape the body, why do other programs such as circuit training, various aerobic activities, and sports fail to reshape the entire body? Let's discuss them one at a time.

Circuit training is done on a "circuit" of machines in a gym, where the exerciser does one set (a group of repetitions) of one exercise for a given body part at a machine or exercise station, and then, without resting, moves to another machine or exercise station, and does one set of an exercise for another body part, and so on, until the circuit is completed. At this point, sometimes the circuit is repeated, but in any case, in total, the exerciser does only a total of one or two sets of an exercise per body part.

Such a system is good for an aerobic effect on the heart and lungs, and is better than nothing when it comes to muscle stimulation, but it can never help to reshape any body part. Why? Because the principle of muscle isolation is ignored—not enough work is done on one body part before moving to the next body part. In addition, the pyramid system is ignored. (And how can one pyramid weights anyway, when one does only one set for a body part?)

Aerobic activities are usually done for twenty or more minutes on various pieces of exercise equipment. Some people mistakenly believe that they can reshape a specific body part by using a piece of aerobic equipment that mainly utilizes that body part. This is a myth.

For example, you can never achieve a perfectly symmetrical, well-defined, muscular upper body by using the rowing machine because you are not using weight in a way that encourages muscle building—you are not using heavy-enough weight—you are not pyramiding the weight, and you are not resting between sets. Also, you are not hitting the muscle from a variety of angles. By doing the repetitive rowing movements, all you can achieve is some upper body strength, the burning of some fat, and increased heart and lung capacity—no small accomplishments in and of themselves, but certainly not the reshaping of the upper body.

The same holds true for any other strictly aerobic workouts. Bike riding, jogging, running, or stair stepping can help to strengthen your hips and thighs, but they can never give you perfect muscularity and definition in those areas.

To try to reshape your body by means of your sport is an exercise in foolishness because any given sport will require concentrated use of one or two body parts and, in essence, neglect other body parts. For example, tennis players have at least one well-developed forearm, swimmers have excellent backs and shoulders, and soccer players have muscular legs. But what about the other body parts? There is simply no way around it. In order to get the ideal body shape, you must work out with weights the right way!

NO MORE WASTED TIME

Perhaps you have spent years trying in vain to combine various techniques that you hoped would give you the body of your dreams, but nothing has worked. You may have improved your heart and lung capacity and burned some fat, but you still have that paunch, and your muscles still don't look the way you want them to look.

Why struggle any longer in vain? The science of how to reshape the body into its most ideal form has already been perfected. There's no need to cast about in desperation. Your search is over.

WHERE DO AEROBICS FIT INTO THIS WORKOUT?

Aerobics are very important for the health of your heart and lungs, and are excellent for burning additional body fat. In addition, aerobics will help you to perform the Top Shape Workout without losing your breath or having to stop for frequent rests. For this reason, I highly recommend that if you have the time, you add aerobics to your routine. You can easily do this either before or after you do your Top Shape Workout, or on the days you're not doing your workout. Various possible workout plans are discussed on pp. 66–68. But in case you don't have time to do aerobics, yet you want an aerobic workout, here's the answer for you.

THE GIANT SET SPEED WORKOUT—IT'S BETTER THAN AEROBICS OR JOGGING

If you choose to do the giant set speed workout, you will in fact kill two birds with one stone. You will work with weights to build muscle and reshape your body, and at the same time keep your heart and lungs within the ideal fat-burning range.

The giant set speed workout allows you to burn maximum fat while shaping your muscles, and it gives you maximum muscle definition, but since you will be using lighter weights in order to cope with the lack of rest time, you will get smaller muscles than those afforded by the regular Top Shape Workout.

This system is ideal for those of you who don't have the extra time to do an aerobic program but wish to be in top shape. It offers the same positive attributes as jogging, for example, and is in fact in many ways more convenient than jogging, because it is done in the privacy of one's own home with a minimum of equipment rather than outside in the cold and/or dark, or on an expensive treadmill. Details about this system are given on pp. 58–59.

In addition, whether you choose the giant set plan or not, the Top Shape Workout will reshape your front and back thighs and calves as well (of course, only if you choose the optional leg workout), whereas jogging only helps to shape your calves.

YOU WON'T LOOK LIKE A BODYBUILDER—YOU WILL CONTROL HOW BIG YOU GET

Believe it or not, some men fear that the minute they pick up a weight they'll turn into Arnold Schwarzenegger. In fact, you would have to lift very heavy weights for hours each day to get to that point. If you don't believe me, go to any hard-core bodybuilding gym, and see the heavy weights those men lift.

What will happen to you if you follow this program (you will be using ten-, fifteen-, and twenty-pound dumbbells for the most part; a little heavier later if you choose), is you will achieve moderate muscularity—muscles tailored to your liking.

As you follow the workout, after, say, a month, if by some miracle your body responds to the weights in such a way that your muscles are getting bigger than you want them to be, you can always switch to the giant set speed workout, which speeds up your workout time and produces somewhat smaller muscles. The fact is, however, that this is unlikely to happen, because even with the hardest work, it is almost impossible to put on more than five to seven pounds of muscle per year.

If, on the other hand, after a few months you decide that you aren't getting big enough, you can always switch to the putting-on-size program (see p. 65). The point is, you never have to worry about something happening to your size. You can control it. You have plenty of time to see in the mirror before anything major happens. You can tailor your muscles to your exact liking as you go along.

WHAT ABOUT GENETICS?

This workout is not designed for the genetically gifted. It is designed for the average or below average. Of course if you are genetically gifted, lucky you. You will get into shape even faster than indicated in the outline in Chapter 2.

Look at the before-and-after men in that chapter. None of them is genetically blessed when it comes to body shape. Yet each of them achieved a degree of fitness that is more than pleasing to the eye. So don't worry about your genetics. This program assumes that you have average or worse genetics.

WHAT MAKES A MAN APPEAR "OLD"?

Other than facial changes, what makes a man begin to appear old? I believe it's the change in muscularity. You see, muscles serve as the antigravity force that keeps your body from hunching over and looking withered. It is well-formed muscles that keep your head up, your shoulders back, and your hips and legs powerful enough to propel your body in an energetic stride. It is strong, well-formed muscles that make for good posture, as opposed to a slumped appearance and a shuffling walk.

REVERSE THE AGING PROCESS AND HAVE A BETTER-SHAPED BODY THAN WHEN YOU WERE AT YOUR PEAK

Aging is the result of atrophy. Every year after thirty, the human body begins to lose a small percentage of muscle and bone density if nothing is done to compensate for that natural attrition process. If, however, something is done to build muscle and bone, not only can naturally lost muscle and bone be replaced, but it can be added to—so that instead of "aging," your body will actually "youthe." In other words, you can have more muscularity and thicker bones in your forties than you did in your twenties.

As muscles are challenged, they will respond. The fact is, if you ask your muscles for more in a gradual manner, they will respond by giving you more—they will grow and be stronger and better shaped and defined. If, on the other hand, you ask your muscles for less (what most people do as they get older), they will respond by giving you less and will eventually become weaker, smaller, and less perfectly shaped and defined. So you see, by working out with weights, you can in fact reverse the aging process.

In other words, if you don't use it, you will lose it. But if you demand that your muscles work, you will not only maintain them, you will increase them, and since you will be using movements designed to give you perfect symmetry, you will also shape them into their ideal form. In fact, your muscles will be better shaped than they were even in your twenties because now you will consciously sculpt them into perfect form, whereas in your twenties, you depended upon your genetic coding as to the shape of your specific muscles. Your symmetry was at the mercy of your genetics. Now you will control your symmetry. "All the women in the office are kidding me," says a fifty-two-year-old insurance broker, with a gleam in his eye, after three months of using this program. "They want to feel my muscles." "My wife tells me to thank you," says a forty-four-year-old stockbroker, with a sly grin, after only six weeks of working out.

WHAT ABOUT BONE?

That muscle can be increased at any age is not news. Medical experts have known it for a long time. Recently, however, it has been proven beyond a shadow of a doubt that bone can be thickened and strengthened at any age. In other words, even osteoporosis can be prevented.[1]

Working out with weights as described in this book increases bone density by placing stress on the bones in isolation. It is the concentrated stress on the bones that causes them to grow thicker and larger. In fact, studies have been done on ninety-year-olds, who before working out with weights were unable to walk without a cane, climb stairs, or even get up from a chair without assistance. In a matter of months, these ninety-year-olds were able to increase bone density and strength to the point that they could do all of these things by themselves.

ADDED MUSCLE ALLOWS YOU TO EAT MORE WITHOUT GETTING FAT

Have you ever wondered why women get fatter than men of equal height and weight, even if they consume exactly the same food and perform the same amount of exercise? The answer is simple. Muscle.

Because of a naturally produced, increased amount of the male hormone testosterone, men naturally develop more muscle on their bodies than do women, and muscle, unlike any other body material, is active twenty-four hours a day. In fact, muscle fibers vibrate slightly, while other body materials such as bone, blood, and water lie stagnant. Adding to those body materials will not speed up your metabolism, but increasing the muscle on your body will.

That muscle increases one's metabolism can be clearly seen on hulking bodybuilders. They can (and in fact must) consume vast amounts of food just to maintain their weight. In other words, the more muscle a man has on his body, the more he must eat, just to maintain those muscles and not lose weight.

Here's how it works. Two men can be sitting in a chair reading a book. One will burn 100 calories in an hour of reading, the other will burn 140 calories in an hour or reading. Why? One man has a much higher percentage of muscle on his body—and since muscle is active as opposed to fat, bone, blood, and other body materials that are stagnant, muscle increases metabolism and causes him to burn more calories even when he is not exercising. It wouldn't matter if he were sleeping, sitting, reading, standing, or walking. If one man has more muscle on his body than another man, all other things being equal, he will burn more calories per hour than the other man.

DIETING ALONE WILL NEVER DO IT

It really depresses me to see how misinformed some men are, and how they actually defeat their own purpose in their efforts to get in shape. A case in point is a gentleman I shall call Joe. He's a businessman who had just turned forty, and proudly announced to me that he weighs the same now as he did when he was twenty-five. "I finally did it," he bragged. "I eat only one meal a day—that's it." (The worst thing he could do, because if you go more than five hours without eating, your metabolism slows down, and you burn less fat.) "I now fit into pants I couldn't wear since college." "Great," I replied. "But are you in shape?" "I guess so," he said. "I run five miles a day and I do a hundred sit-ups." Then I asked him to show me a photograph of himself at twenty-five, and one of him now—in a bathing suit. He dug them up.

When we looked at the photographs together, before I could say a word, his face dropped. Since the earlier photo, his muscles had shrunken visibly. He was not happy with what he saw. Chances are, not only did his muscles shrink from the normal muscle atrophy that happens every year after thirty, but from the starvation dieting that he was doing. (If you cut your calorie intake to below 1,000 to 1,500, depending upon your size, your body will use muscle as fuel for energy as well as fat.) Joe's previously well-rounded, muscular shoulders now sloped slightly downward and his massive chest had sunk. His formerly strong neck looked scrawny, and his athletic-looking V shape was gone due to atrophy of his back (latissimus dorsi) muscles. In addition, he had small rolls of fat on his lower back. His formerly muscular arms were now too thin—and in fact reminded me of a woman's arms in some respects. His previously "ripped" stomach had changed too (see p. 45). The upper abdominal area was almost flat, with no definition, and he now sported a little pouch of fat in the lower area, and he had little love handles on his sides. His formerly well-shaped thighs now reminded me of chicken legs. In his twenties, Joe looked handsomely muscular. Now, at forty, at that same weight, he appeared to be sadly frail, and in some areas, fat. But he couldn't see it until he looked at the two photographs of himself—side by side.

Why did this happen? His body composition had shifted. He had dieted to keep his weight down, but he had lost muscle naturally over the years. In addition, he had gained body fat. The end result, even though he weighed the same, he certainly did not look the same. In discussing the earlier photograph in contrast to his present look, I tried to convince him that he had to work out with weights in order to build muscles and regain, and even better, the body of his youth. "I don't want to gain weight," he said. (He had heard that muscles weigh more than fat, and they do.) "What's the difference what the scale says?" I asked. "Isn't what you see in the mirror more important?" "I don't want to have to buy new suits," he protested. Nothing I said could convince him that he would not gain massive amounts of weight, and that by the time he started getting muscle, he would even welcome having to buy a larger jacket if he should be so lucky as to put on that much muscle. The man would not do it. He had made up his mind. He was afraid to try weights, and for him, the case was closed.

There are so many men who even in this day and age are as misinformed as Joe. Many of them have written to me, asking for help, because nothing they have tried has worked. Fortunately, most of the men have open minds, and are now working with this program, and will soon have before-and-after photographs of their own to show.

YOU WILL INCREASE YOUR STRENGTH AND HAVE IMPROVED ABILITY IN SPORTS

In addition to all of the above, working out as described in this program will increase your overall strength, and in turn, improve your performance in your favored sport. How so? If all characteristics are the same (skill, speed, age, and so forth), it is the stronger sportsman who will defeat the weaker. Why? Because when a muscle is strong, it is able to put forth more intense effort. In other words, it can do more work in the same amount of time, or do equal work in less time. So if you do the Top Shape Workout your muscles will not only become stronger, they will also enable your body to move faster.

THIS PROGRAM BENEFITS YOUR MIND AND ATTITUDE

With all of the advantages to health and body, one might be surprised to hear that it is perhaps the mind that benefits the most from this workout. A whole chapter is devoted to this subject (Chapter 3), but for now, let me say that you will notice that you are generally more alert and relaxed once you start this program. The workout literally "wakes you up," and at the same time, provides a release of physical tension. Your attitude changes. You don't take things in such a life-and-death manner as before, and in fact, your sense of humor is unleashed. Your self-confidence builds. You find yourself willing to take chances in your business and personal life that you were previously afraid to take. You may decide to go for some evening classes—to reach for a promotion, or even to change jobs. You may take up a new sport. You think: "I was able to take control of my body and I see the tangible results in front of me—I can take control of other situations too. I can make changes there!" Anything can happen once you get in shape. You'll be amazed.

Notes:

1. Dr. Sydney Bonnic, director of Osteoporosis Services, Cooper Clinic, cited this study to John Stossel of ABC News on *20/20*, May 10, 1991. The study is mentioned on pp. 7–9 of the *Journal Graphics* transcript.

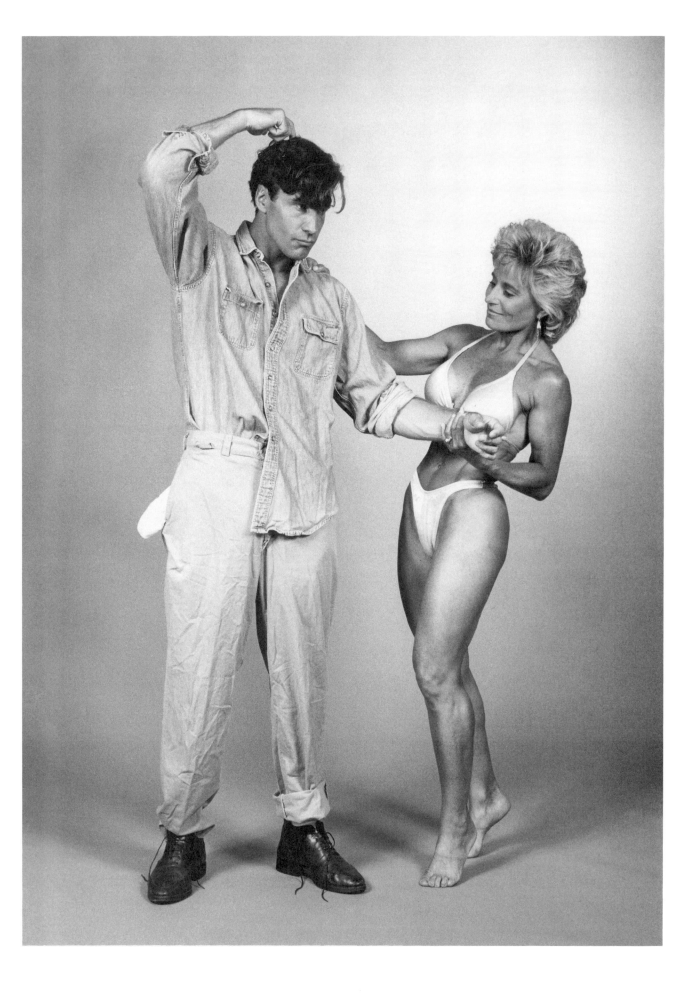

2

Good Shape—From Before to After

Right now you must be saying, "I wonder how long it will take me to get into top shape!" It will not take you as long as you may think. You'll have the body of your dreams in twelve to twenty-four weeks. The before-and-after men in this chapter did it, and so can you.

If your body is not in its top shape—its most perfect form—you're actually in a better position than a top athlete or champion bodybuilder who had achieved the peak of fitness in his youth—and now cannot possibly improve on his body. As time goes by, he can only hope to maintain it, or to watch it go downhill. You, on the other hand, can experience the excitement of looking better and better as you go along, and of eventually achieving a more fit and attractive physique than when you were at what you used to think was your best.

With this program, the more out of shape you are, the better—because the more dramatic will be the changes that you will see and feel. In fact, even if you are well into your forties, fifties, sixties, or older, you will look and feel young again.

An interesting study was conducted by a group of scientists. Men who were over sixty and in top shape, and men who were in their twenties and who were badly out of shape were compared in terms of physical strength, agility, and muscularity. The researchers could not tell that the men over sixty were older than the men in their twenties. In fact, the testing indicated that the men in their twenties were the "old" men.[1] The point is, it's not what age does to your body, but what *you* do to your body as you age that is most important.

It's easy to understand how this principle works if you think in terms of what happens to a body part if it is left in a cast for six weeks—it atrophies. But once you start to use that body part again, it comes back to shape. If you've ever had a cast on your arm, you know exactly what I'm talking about. When you first take the cast off, your arm is thin and shriveled because of immobilization, but after a few weeks of using it again, the arm returns to normal. It works the same way with the Top Shape Workout—only better. With this program, not only will you use muscles that you used before but gradually neglected, you will also challenge other muscles that you never really exercised properly—so by the time you are finished, your entire body will be in balance and near-perfect symmetry—and will look better than it did before—even when you were at your best.

FORGET ABOUT BODY TYPES

We've all heard about body types. There is the traditional mesomorphic (a tendency toward muscular, ideal in shape and size), the endomorphic (a tendency toward fat), and ectomorphic (a tendency toward leanness).

Body types only exist in the before stage—not in the after stage. How can this be? Although you may have a leaning toward a certain body type before you start working out, once you have used the program for twelve or more weeks, your body shape will have evolved away from its original state and into the more ideal mesomorphic form. So forget about body types. It doesn't matter what your genetic tendency is. You'll overcome it with this program. Take a look at the before-and-after men. I'll bet you would label them one body type before and a different body type after!

THE SHAPE YOU'RE IN

Let's talk about the shape you are in now. Chances are, either you are overweight and out of shape, the right weight but out of shape, or too thin or hollow and out of shape. In addition, if you are well into your thirties or older, you have also begun to experience muscle atrophy. (By the time a man is sixty-five years old, unless he does something about it, he will have lost 50 percent of the muscle he had when he was eighteen years old.) Take a look at the following categories and decide where you stand right now.

Fat and Out of Shape

Take a look at Dave. He's fifty-four years old and thirty-five pounds overweight in his before photo. In his after photo, six months later, he's lost thirty-five pounds of fat, but he's gained about two and a half pounds of muscle! He used to weigh himself every week, agonizing over the scale and worrying about not only his general health, but his blood pressure. Now he never weighs himself (the mirror is his new scale), and he has been given a clean bill of health by his company doctor. His blood pressure has gone down from 155 over 115 to normal.

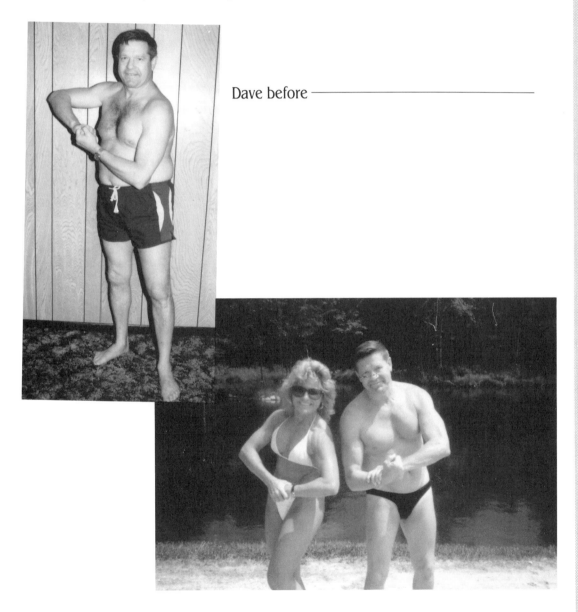

Dave before ————————————————————

Dave after six months ————————————————

Now let's look at Pat. At forty-seven and a half years old, he looked like, in his own words, "an old man." After following the low-fat eating plan (see Chapter 9) for six months (he lost thirty-five pounds) and doing the workout for only three months ("I know I should have started the workout at the same time I started the diet, but I needed some time to get psyched," he confesses), he not only looks younger and feels healthier, but sexier too! And his wife, Cynthia, says, "And he acts sexier too."

Pat can now be seen on the ski slopes, accomplishing feats in skiing that he dared not try fifteen years ago. The workout has helped him to improve in all of his sports, and he has taken to showing off his body at every available occasion. "For the first time in his life, he wears tank tops," his wife Cynthia says. "He even wears them to the store when we go shopping."

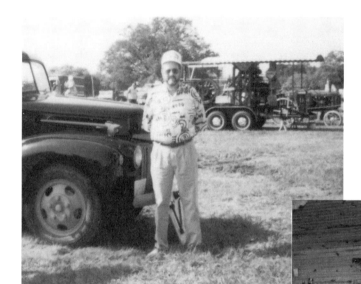

Pat before ————

Pat after three months ————

Kevin before ———————

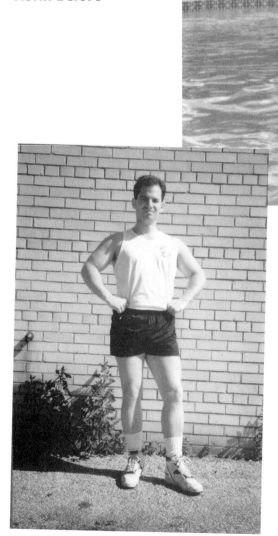

Kevin after six months ———————

Kevin weighed 220 pounds in his before photo. He was fat and getting fatter every day. "I gained sympathy weight while my wife was pregnant," he says. Finally, he decided to start the workout and the low-fat eating plan.

It took him six months to lose the excess fat and replace it with hard-earned muscle. At thirty years old he is a healthy 175 pounds. He says: "I'm glad I decided to get in shape instead of going over the hill before my time. You can't put a price on this workout and eating plan."

The Right Weight and Out of Shape

Look at Augustine. He is thirty-four years old in his before photo. He's neither fat nor skinny—in fact, if you use your imagination, I'm sure you can see that he would not appear overweight at all in a suit. What's wrong with him? His muscles are not well developed or well defined, and he doesn't have symmetry (his muscles are not placed over his body in a balanced way). In addition, even though he is not overweight, he is carrying some extra fat in his abdominal area—a favorite place in men for storing excess fat.

Augustine didn't lose any weight in three months' time; in fact, he gained a pound and a half—obviously of pure muscle. But you can clearly see that now he looks a lot better—having placed just the right-sized muscles all over his body.

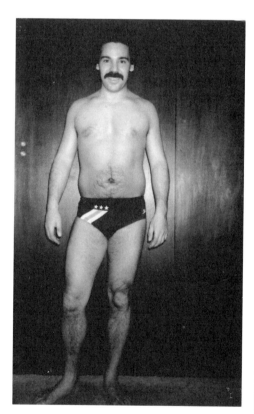

Augustine before ——————————————

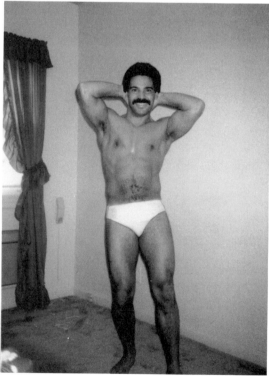

Augustine after three months ——————

Too Thin and Out of Shape

Stephen is forty-five years old in his before photograph. He is too thin, but it's more than that. In his own words, he is "hollow." His muscles are underdeveloped from a combination of disuse and natural atrophy over time. Stephen didn't take the time to shoot a special before photo when he started the program, in his late forties, but look at him now, at forty-nine after six months of training. His muscles have filled out—he no longer looks hollow. He has developed his trapezius muscles, rounded out and defined his shoulders, built up and defined his chest, defined his abdominals and removed the excess fat, and clearly developed his arms. Stephen now has such a well-balanced body that you would think he were a model.

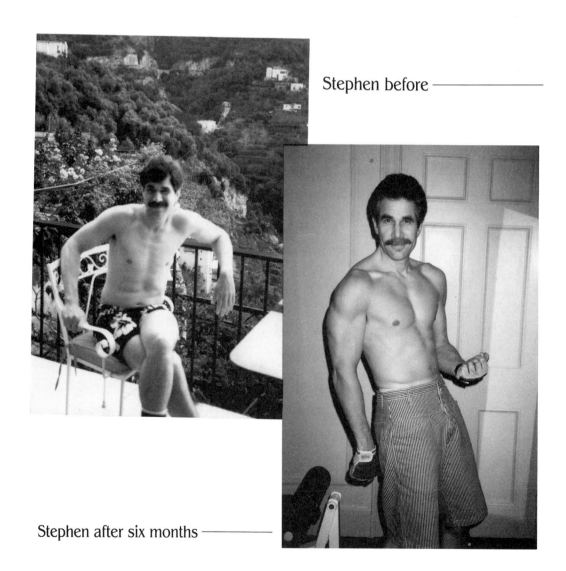

Stephen before ⸺

Stephen after six months ⸺

21

Wow! Look What Graham Did in Only Four Weeks

Now take a look at Graham. He's thirty-five years old, and has only been working out for four weeks! Notice the reduced gut, and what to me is even more impressive in such a short amount of time, the increased muscularity of his entire upper body—chest, shoulders, back, and arms. "I've gone from jellyfish to shark in one cycle of the moon," says Graham. "Most people become lean and mean when they start working out," says his wife, Kathleen. "In Graham's case, he's become lean and happy—and he's gone down from a thirty-six to a thirty-three pants size! That makes *me* very happy."

Graham before ———————

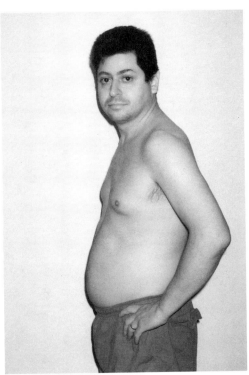

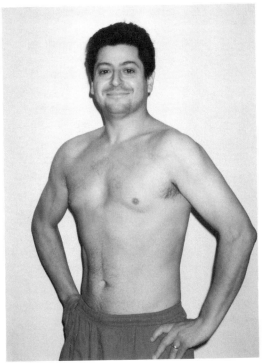

Graham after four weeks ———————

WHAT CAN YOU EXPECT, WEEK BY WEEK, UNTIL YOU REACH YOUR GOAL?

What will happen once you start working out? No matter what shape you're in, fat and out of shape, the right weight and out of shape, or too thin and out of shape, you can expect certain changes week by week and month by month.

One Week

Your first week of training will be the most challenging because that's when you'll experience most of your soreness, even if you do break in gently—and so much more if you don't. One fellow confesses: "I didn't break in gently, but instead did the whole workout the first day. I was in so much pain the next day—and by the following day, when I was supposed to work out again, I almost didn't do it. Then I remembered that if you work through the soreness, the workout would be like a massage for my muscles. In blind faith I forced myself to do it, and sure enough I felt a little better afterward. By the end of the week the soreness was about half, and in another week, there was almost no soreness at all."

Another problem in week one will be thoughts of self-doubt. But those doubts will be quickly dispelled when you start to look better and feel more energy. "When I could hardly do a crunch with my big belly in the way," says one man, "I started wondering if this could work for me. But then by the end of the week, my skin coloring had improved and people were telling me I looked healthier. I also have more energy. I used to come home from work and nap. Now I go straight to the weights and work out. It's worth it. I'm glad I got through the first week."

Two Weeks

By your second week, you'll start to become more familiar with the exercises, so the workout will flow with much more ease. "I'm going through the workout much faster now—I don't have to look at the photographs as much," says one man.

You'll also begin to feel stronger, and your body will be harder to the touch. "I've already upped some of my weights, my body told me to do it," says one man. "I don't see much of a difference in my shape yet, but my whole body feels harder. I know something is happening."

You may even begin to see a difference in your sport at this early stage. A man in his fifties told me, "I was playing basketball and a kid was running into me, so I got into a defensive position. It felt like he was running into a stone wall. He asked me, 'What did you do?' The truth is, I don't know what I did. I just felt stronger."

Three Weeks

By now you'll be used to the routine and you'll hardly ever have to refer to the book. Those of you who are overweight will have lost up to six pounds of fat (the scale may show a greater loss because you may have been retaining water). You will begin to see muscle development and definition in some areas, depending on which of your body parts respond most quickly.

"I can't believe it but I see development in my chest," says one man. "I can actually see a difference in my shoulders, I feel like I have shoulder pads on," says another man. "Before I hated looking in the mirror, now I'm wearing the mirrors out. All you have to do is see one little muscle and you can't look at it enough," says a third man.

You'll begin to walk, sit, and stand with more energy and bounce. "My posture has improved. Now I throw my shoulders back when I walk—and instead of slumping down in my chair, I sit up. This is amazing," says one of the before-and-after men.

Four Weeks

You will see subtle and not-so-subtle changes all over your body in four weeks. Your chest, shoulders, biceps, triceps, back, and abdominals will begin to show definition and development. (If you are still more than ten pounds overweight, your abdominal area will not show much definition, because your developing muscles will still be hidden by a coating of fat, but your stomach will feel harder.) Your calves (if you have chosen to exercise your legs) will begin to develop, and you will begin to feel strength in your thighs and you will see some definition.

"My biceps have definitely gotten bigger and I feel muscles in my stomach I never thought I had," says one man. "I can actually flex my triceps, and feel something," says another. "I swear I can see traps developing, but isn't it too soon for that?" says a third.

Others will begin to notice the change. "People are starting to comment all the time on how good I look," says one man. "I'm walking around the office with my shoulders back—like a jock."

Eight Weeks

You will continue to see muscle development and definition all over your body. The more difficult body parts will begin to show development—and your lats will begin to widen, giving your waist a smaller appearance. Your stomach will continue to show definition. Your biceps will become more rounded and defined, and your triceps will have more definition. Your shoulders will increase in fullness and you will begin to see definition in your rear deltoids (back shoulder area). Your chest will continue to fill out, and those of you who previously suffered from "pencil necks" will be encouraged by the development of your trapezius muscles.

"I'm glad you told me to pose, because when I do a lat spread, I can really see a difference now," says one man. "When I flex my stomach, I can really see my abs coming in," says another.

You will also get stronger. By now, those of you who weren't able to handle the ten-, fifteen-, and twenty-pound dumbbells will be able to use them for most exercises with ease. Some of you will have increased your weights two or three times by now. All of you will be stronger.

Your improved appearance will become more and more noticeable. "I'm starting to look so much better—people at work are commenting—and that makes me feel better about myself. On an executive level, it's really important not only to feel good, but to look good too," says one man.

Those of you who are overweight will continue to lose weight—up to sixteen pounds. The waist of your pants will be swimming on you, but you may find that your jacket is getting a little snug from the muscles you are developing on your upper body.

You will also continue to experience higher and higher energy levels. "Since I've been working out, my adrenaline is flowing—I'm more lively. I'm in high gear," says one man.

Twelve Weeks

When you look in the mirror, your body will appear to have been completely reshaped. You will not believe that it was possible to have done so much in so little time. In fact, by now everyone you know will be asking you for your secret, and when you tell them what it is, they won't believe you. You'll find yourself trying to explain it all day long—and you'll have people asking you to help them get started. Sometimes you'll wish they would leave you alone.

At this point, because of the dramatic changes in most of your body parts, some of you will notice "lagging body parts." Your biceps and triceps may be perfect in your eyes, but your chest may still need a little work; or your chest may be fine, but your lats may still be too narrow. Everyone has a different genetic makeup. Some men develop shoulders seemingly overnight, while others have to struggle for months to see any major changes. Others seem to develop instant chests, while others battle endlessly to build that area.

You will soon find out which of your body parts respond most quickly, and which body parts tend to lag behind. You should continue to do the regular workout at this point, except, if you wish, you can add in the "Bombs Away" program found in one of my previous books, *Gut Busters*, for your abdominal area. Your other body parts may "come in" in another twelve weeks. At that point, if you're still not satisfied, you can apply some of the special techniques found on pp. 62–64.

Those of you who are overweight will have lost up to twenty-four pounds—but since you will have also put on some muscle (muscle weighs more than fat), the scale may not show such a dramatic loss. By now you will begin to willingly give up using the scale as your measure, because you will come to realize that what you see in the mirror is the real measure.

Twenty-four Weeks

Now your body will be close to its most perfect form. In short, you will be looking good, and everyone will notice it. Your new body will by now have had a dramatic effect on your mind. You may find yourself going back to school to take some courses or beginning a new sport. "I joined a karate class," says one man. "I'm finishing my law degree," says another. "I've quit my job and gotten a better one," says a third. "My wife had left me and I was depressed all the time," said another. "But now that I've been working out, I have more dates than I can handle. It's not just my body. I know that. It's my attitude. I feel good about myself, and women pick up on that. No one wants to be around a depressed person."

Your clothing style will change. "When I told my girlfriend that I was going to give up my boxer-short-type bathing suit for a bathing suit that shows more, she almost fell over. But she liked the look once I put on the suit." "I never thought I would wear tank tops to the gym," says another man. "All I had was a bunch of old T-shirts with holes in them. Now you see me in the store buying all kinds of new stuff."

Your body will look so good that at times you won't be able to deal with it yourself. "If you would have told me six months ago that I could have this body, I would never have believed you," says one man. "It's really surprising what you can do if you follow a routine and stick with it. People have been saying, 'I can't believe it.' They see muscles right through my clothes."

Those of you who were extremely overweight will have lost up to forty-eight pounds. If you have more to go, as you continue the low-fat eating plan and the workout, in time you will lose all of your excess body fat. As you get closer to your goal, your body will naturally start to give up its weight more slowly—you may lose only a pound or less a week. But it won't matter. You won't even care what the scale says. The mirror will tell you all that you need to know.

As Time Goes By

As time goes by—in nine months, in a year—you'll see subtle improvements in your body. Your lagging body parts will show some improvement, even if you don't use special techniques. You'll have more thickness (mass) and more definition.

You can continue to use this workout forever, and you will maintain your body. But if at any point you want to change your body—to make it fuller or more defined—you can take advantage of the methods on pp. 62–65.

In any case, instead of losing muscle and appearing to get older and older, you will maintain, consolidate, and refine your muscle, and in fact appear to get younger and younger.

Your weight will eventually stabilize, and the last thing on your mind, except for idle curiosity, will be "How much do I weigh?" If you were previously obsessed with dieting, you will be free of that too. You'll be eating and exercising for your body, and it will be fun rather than punishment because you will feel as if you are "in training," and you won't want to break that training. (More about eating in Chapter 9.)

Notes:
1. John Jerome, *Staying With It* (New York: Viking Press, 1985) p. 60.

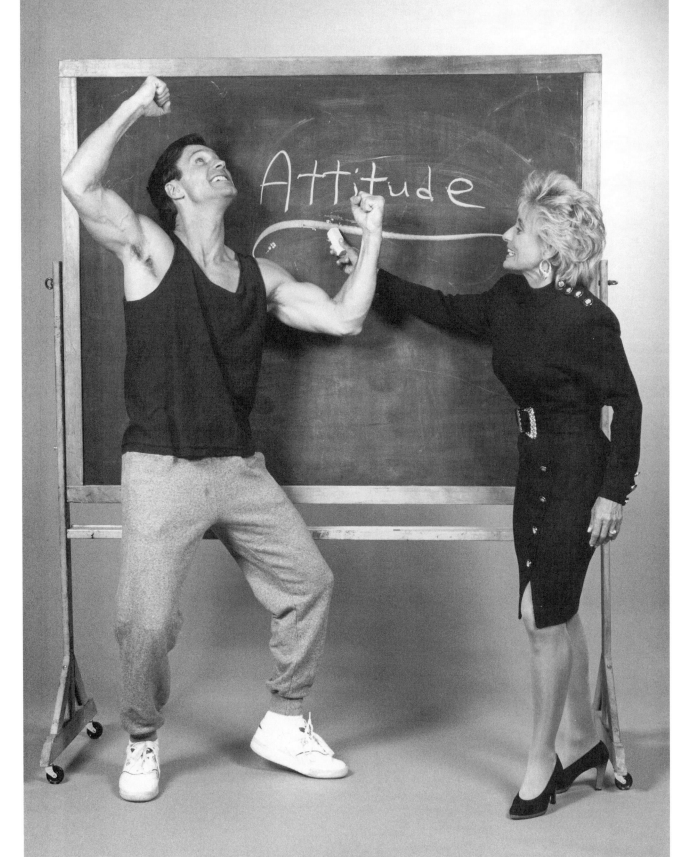

3

Mind Shape

To a great extent the mind controls the body. For example, it is the mind that ultimately decides whether or not to listen to the body when the body says, "I'm too tired to get up now. I want to sleep another hour." It is the mind that says yes or no when the body cries, "I don't feel like working out, I'd rather relax and watch TV." It is the mind that gives the okay or the refusal when the body declares, "I want that greasy hamburger."

There will always be a battle between the body and the mind—but in the end, it is the mind that has the ultimate say. This, in fact, is very good news. It means that you have the assurance that if *you decide* that you want this—that you want to be in top shape, and that you are going to pay the small, yet very real price, you *will* achieve your goal.

THE POWER OF THE HUMAN WILL

What is the human will? Is it the mind? No. It's more than the mind. I believe it is the soul. It has its own energy and enthusiasm. It's that part of yourself that rises up when called upon and refuses to let you be compromised. It is the part of you that you use to direct your life. Your will gives you the power of self-control in the face of even the most compelling temptations. Time and again, you decide whether or not to use that power to resist temptation and "stay the course," the course that you have decided is best for you, whether it be a career decision, a relationship decision, or a commitment to your body.

When you come to think about it, it is your will that has gotten you to where you are now in your life. The measure of your success is the measure of your will, and how you have used it. It is what makes deliberate and conscious decisions for you, time and time again.

It is your will that will save you when you are tempted to skip a workout: it is what will remind you of your purpose and intention, and give you the resolve to follow through. In fact, time and again, when your body says no, your will will say, "Do it," because your will has the power to control your actions. It can order you to do what you have determined to do. In fact, after exerting your will over your body for a few months, your body will seem to be hypnotized by your will. Soon your body will go on "automatic," and do what is expected, except on occasion, when you (your will) will have to remind it of who is in charge.

MAKING THE COMMITMENT: THE BENEFITS VERSUS THE COST

But in order for the above to happen, you must first make the commitment. You must decide how important it is to you to, once and for all, get your body into its top shape. In order to do this, you must weigh the benefits against the cost, and see whether or not it is worth it to you. Let's do that right now. First, let's look at the benefits, then we'll count the cost.

The Benefits

Improved Self-Image and Self-Esteem. Stand in front of a full-length mirror and take a hard look at yourself—do it right now—don't change your clothing. Does your body tell the truth about you—or does it give a wrong impression? If your body has gotten out of shape, if your muscles have been neglected, and if fat has taken over certain areas of your body, chances are your body misrepresents who you really are.

You are clearly not your body, yet your body says something about you. You may, in fact, be a very strong-willed, self-determined, successful man in many areas of life—yet your body may imply that you are not strong, not in control. You have been able to succeed despite your body, but in fact, up until now, your body has not been a help to your self-image or your self-esteem, but rather a hindrance, an obstacle that you have had to overcome.

If you get your body into shape, instead of being a hindrance to you, an obstacle to be overcome, your body will be a help to you—visual proof that you are strong and determined. Just looking at your improved body will send you a message every time. It will remind you that you are in control. It will reflect the strength of your will. You will in fact think better of yourself (self-esteem is, in fact, your reputation with yourself, or what you think of yourself). In short, you self-esteem will permanently improve.

Improved Career Opportunities and Personal Life. When self-image and self-esteem have improved, along with a very real improvement in the physical body, things can also improve career-wise, because you project a different image to those around you, and because your own idea of who you are has changed.

You will begin to ask for, and get more in a job situation, because you will believe that you deserve it, and those with whom you deal will come to see you in a different light. For example, if you are seeking a promotion on the job, you'll be more likely to believe that you deserve it, and in fact, you'll be perceived by your superiors as more worthy of it.

Your improved self-esteem will cause you to think in terms of doing more with your life in general. I've seen men change jobs for better jobs, go back to school to finish degrees, and even go into their own business after getting into shape. The discipline involved in the program teaches you an unconscious lesson. "I can make things happen," you think. "I was successful in reshaping my body, I have the power to handle other difficult things. I can make changes here too," you say. "I'm a fine-looking fellow," you think. "I deserve better than this," you conclude.

I've seen men take up new sports, get out of negative relationships, make new friends, take long-dreamed-of vacations, and in general, begin to live life to the fullest, after getting in shape. I've seen men who were previously dour in nature open up and let their sense of humor have its way. In fact, I've seen men transformed before my very eyes once they have gotten their body into the shape that reflects the person they really are inside.

Increased Energy. After you have passed the initial break-in stage (one to three weeks), working out in and of itself will cause you to feel more energetic for hours after the workout, due to the increased blood circulation and muscle stimulation. But there's more to it than that. Once you begin to get in shape, your muscles and bones will have more strength, and this will give you permanent energy, because it won't take as much effort to do what you used to do before. You'll walk with more gusto. You'll even sit and stand differently. You'll get more done in a day without as much effort.

People will notice. "What's different about you?" they'll ask, even though they can't really see your muscles under your suit. Just watch and see. Every one of the before-and-after men told me that people said similar things to them. And the men smile—thinking, "Yes. Something is different. Something big is happening."

Improved Health. When you neglect things, they deteriorate. If you don't keep your home in good repair, when you go to sell it, it becomes a "handyman special." If you don't change the oil on your car regularly, you ruin the engine. If you neglect to exercise your body, it deteriorates, not only externally, but internally. Working out and eating the diet described in this program can remedy years of neglect.

Your blood pressure will go down, your cholesterol level will go down, your bones will get thicker, and your blood circulation—and in turn your skin tone—will improve. And, if you follow the giant set speed workout or you do the optional aerobics, in addition, your resting heart rate will go down, and you'll be able to walk faster, or even run without getting out of breath.

Every one of the before-and-after men in Chapter 2 has told me that the above has happened to them—and what's more, they have medical records to prove it. There's really no mystery in it. Medical science is in agreement. The results are inevitable. Your health will improve if you work out sensibly with weights, reduce your fat and cholesterol intake to healthful levels, and engage in moderate aerobic activities.

Relieves Stress and Clears the Mind. "I start my workout with a million problems on my mind," says one of the before-and-after men. "I can even consciously be worrying about how I'm going to pull off a big business transaction, but after a few minutes, in spite of myself, I've forgotten all about business and I'm concentrating on the workout. Thirty minutes later, when I'm getting dressed, it's as if the cobwebs have cleared—and the tension is gone. The workout has relieved my stress to the point where I have relaxed enough to see a solution I may never have seen otherwise."

Restores Youth. As discussed on pp. 9–10, every year after thirty, muscle and bone slightly deteriorate. In fact, experts say that by the age of sixty-five, unless a man does something to reverse it, he will have lost up to fifty percent of his muscle, and beginning at age fifty, men lose .04 percent bone per year.

But more than health and youth—the restoration of needed muscle and bone—the workout restores the look of youth. It makes the body look more appealing than it did in its youth, because the workout is based upon the bodyshaping principles of champion bodybuilders, who know how to create the perfectly symmetrical body. In fact, you can and will have a more balanced-looking, well-shaped body than you had when you were at your peak—but before you worked out with a plan such as this.

Relaxed Confidence. Instead of continually worrying about your body and your health, you'll be able to lay the issue to rest once and for all, and devote your energy to other things. Your body shape and your health will be under control, and you'll have peace of mind in that area. No longer will you have to spend time searching for ways to get in shape. That will be out of the way. Now, you will be able to save your energy for advancing your career and achieving your goals in life, or just for relaxing and enjoying your newfound fitness.

The Cost

This section is going to be strangely brief. The cost is: two hours a week (either three forty-minute sessions; or four thirty-minute sessions).

When you think of the benefits, and weigh them against the cost, ask yourself the question: Is it worth it? Is it worth two hours a week for what I will get in return? I think your answer will be yes. It's worth it.

MAKE PLANS

Where will you get this thirty to forty minutes three to four days a week? Your schedule may be so busy, you may not be able to take it from television time because perhaps you don't even watch TV, and you may not even be able to take it from socializing time—because you don't even have time for that. Well, if it comes down to it, I dare say, it's worth it to take it from sleep time, or even your lunchtime.

You may want to work out first thing in the morning—whether at home or in the gym. It's really the best idea to just pop out of bed, go to the bathroom, and then without further ado hit the bench and dumbbells and begin the workout. Thirty to forty minutes later, it's over. You can brush your teeth, take a shower, eat a light breakfast, and go to work. It would be out of the way, and all day long you'd feel great about knowing that you already worked out. You would also have more energy for the day.

If you're already getting up at 5:00 A.M. or earlier, and you simply won't give up one more moment of sleep, your next best bet is to work out lunchtime. If there is no gym nearby, convince your boss to allow you a space for a bench and three sets of dumbbells. Many employers are now aware of the benefits of physical fitness and will be glad to comply. In fact, you can volunteer to start a program for others in your office, and your boss may be delighted with your offer.

The next possibility is, after work, either to go straight to a gym, or to go home and before you do anything else, put on your shorts and T-shirt and go to your bench and dumbbells and work out. If you don't live alone, engage the cooperation of those living in your house. Ask them to let you have thirty minutes for your workout—and then you will be one hundred percent available to them. Most people will cooperate when they see how important it is to you—and even if they fight you at first, after they see how great you start to look and feel, they will in fact probably ask if they can join you.

If you are a traveling man, don't worry. There is a special chapter (8) on how to keep up the workout with little or no equipment—anywhere in the world.

USING YOUR MIND TO SPEED UP YOUR PROGRESS

One of the before-and-after men said: "I think you could be a brainless wonder and go through this workout, and still make progress, even if you never visualized, concentrated, or did any of that psychological stuff. I just do my workout and forget about it—and it works anyway."

The gentleman is right. Even if you did not employ a single one of the techniques offered in the following paragraphs, if you followed the workout, you would still get into shape—because the workout is based upon physical science. Your muscles have to grow and become reshaped if you follow the plan. However, if you do employ the following techniques, you can speed up your progress. They can only add to your success.

Concentrate! To concentrate is to focus on or to direct toward a center. When you are working out, you should direct your mind toward your working muscle—making it the focus, the center of your concentration. Look at the working muscle as you move the dumbbell up and down. Think about the progress it is making. Add to that. Actually "tell" that muscle to grow, and picture in your mind the shape and size you want it to be. Follow strict form. Willfully flex and stretch the muscle with each repetition. Make sure that the muscle you are supposed to be working is actually doing the work!

In order to help you with your concentration, take a good look at the anatomy chart and muscle descriptions on pp. 47–51. Locate each muscle on your own body. True, you may already be well aware of the existence of your biceps muscle, but what about your front, side, and rear deltoid (shoulder) muscles, your trapezius and latissimus dorsi (back) muscles, and so on? If you take the time to clearly locate each of the muscles in the anatomy photographs on pp. 49–50 on your own body, when you work out, you will be able to concentrate with that much more ease.

Help yourself by heading off situations that would interfere with concentration. If you work out at home, make it known that you are not to be disturbed until your workout is over. If you live alone, unplug the phone or put on the answering machine. If necessary, play your music loud to block out any street noises, or the sound of the doorbell.

If you work out in a gym, don't fall into the trap of talking to other men, or waiting around for certain equipment to become available. If someone wants to talk to you, tell him or her, "I'm training for something. I'll talk to you later." They'll think you are a bodybuilder and respect your concentration. If someone is monopolizing a piece of equipment, do another exercise in that muscle group, or ask if you can "work in."

One of the men who works out in the gym says, "I line up my three sets of dumbbells by a flat/incline bench. Then I can go through my whole chest routine, or shoulder routine, or whatever I'm doing for that day. People don't usually interrupt once you have your equipment, and once you look serious." If that doesn't work for you, however, and someone tries to take a piece of the equipment you have lined up, just say, "I'm giant-setting" (and you may well be if you choose the giant set speed workout). If you're in a bodybuilding gym, they'll know what you're talking about and leave you alone. If you're not, they'll probably still leave you alone—they'll assume that you are doing something important and won't want to disturb you.

Remember, the more intense your workout, the more you get out of it. Every time you take a minute to talk or wait, you decrease the efficacy of the workout. You also waste time. Your goal is to get in and out of there—fast. You can always socialize later.

Set a Target Date and Mark It on the Calendar. You will transform your entire body in twelve to twenty-four weeks. You can decide how much time you want to give yourself to achieve this goal. Think carefully. Get a sense of your own timing. Then look at the calender and pick a date anywhere from twelve to twenty-four weeks from your start date. This will be your target date. Circle it on the calendar. Then let your unconscious mind guide you to your goal. If you've picked the maximum time, twenty-four weeks, realize that in about six months the time would have gone by anyway, and had you done nothing your body would either be in the same shape it is now or worse. So don't be impatient with yourself. Twenty-four weeks is nothing when you think of a lifetime of fitness.

Use Your Unconscious Mind. The unconscious mind is like a combination of a computer and a homing torpedo. Once you give your unconscious mind the target date, it will, like the homing torpedo, cause you to zigzag around obstacles to get you to your goal on time. Your unconscious mind will compel you to do a workout when you are tempted to skip one. It will help you to resist eating fatty foods when you are ready to let down your guard. It will urge you on when you are feeling lazy or discouraged. Your unconscious mind is a very powerful tool. Once you clearly state your goal, and give your unconscious mind a target date, it will force you to achieve that goal, even if you try to fight it.

Bodybuilders use this trick all the time. About six months before a contest, they will tell their bodies to look a certain way on contest date, and invariably, their bodies come into that exact form on that date. They program their minds, and their minds deliver the goods.

Take a Before Photo, Visualize in Front of the Mirror, and Pose. It is very important that you take a before photograph of yourself—because if you don't, later, when your entire body has been reshaped, you will have no proof of the dramatic change. Time and again people have written to me lamenting the fact that they didn't take the time to take such a photo. Take the photo. In fact, while you're at it, take a front, side, and rear view. Then hide the photos somewhere—under a desk blotter, for example. Then forget about them for twelve to twenty-four weeks, depending upon the target date you have set. Later, you can join the other before-and-after men in Chapter 2 by pasting your photographs in the allotted space, or you can send some copies to me and who knows, you may be featured in one of my future books!

Have a mental picture of what you want your body to look like. You can look through men's magazines, or dig up an old photograph of yourself when you were in shape—and then draw over it with a felt tip pen to make yourself look even better. Or, you may want to take two identical before photographs. Hide one, and draw over the other with a felt tip pen—making your body look exactly the way you want it to look. Keep that retouched photograph available.

Whenever you catch a view of yourself in the mirror, instead of putting yourself down mentally, or ignoring what you see, take advantage of the opportunity. Picture your body the way it will look on target date. Tell your body to evolve into that form. Believe that you can do it and you will. In the words of Vince Lombardi, former coach of the Green Bay Packers, "Winning is 75 percent mental."[1]

Finally, try some posing. Yes. As fat and out of shape as you may be at the moment, after you have worked out for about two weeks, get a copy of *Muscle and Fitness* magazine, and copy a few of the poses of the muscle men. If you don't want to do that, try posing like the men in Chapter 2. Do a side chest shot like Dave, or an abs shot like Augustine. These men thought I was out of my mind when I first suggested that they pose. In fact, they only did it in the privacy of their bathrooms at first. But after they began to get in shape, they were posing all over the place.

Posing in this sense is not, as you might at first think, a vain and foolish activity. It helps to give you a sense of your muscularity, and it forces you to see that your muscles really do exist, and are in fact beginning to come alive. Posing inspires you to move toward your goal. It helps you to see that you are beginning to look better than you did before, because when you pose, you flex your muscles, forcing them to appear bigger, harder, and more defined. "Posing made me want to try even harder," says one of the men. "It got me excited."

Purchase some muscle magazines. Keep a folder of your favorite poses and whenever you are in the mood, try them out.

Keep Getting Up! No matter how good your intentions, in the beginning you may have a few setbacks. You may start the workout and do it for two or three days, and then something may come up and you'll be forced to skip a few days. You may then think, "Forget it. I'll never do this." Stop the music. Instead, forgive yourself and simply begin again.

It takes time to establish a habit. Reread the benefits section of this chapter. Reinspire yourself. No matter how many times you fall, get up again. Think of it as the difficult beginning stages of something that will eventually become automatic. Remember when you were taught to ride a two-wheeler. You probably took a lot of spills before you could practically ride in your sleep.

Reject Negative Thinking and Talking. People have become ill and even died just because they *thought* they had ingested poison, when in fact they had ingested a harmless food.[2] Your thoughts are powerful. Don't allow negative thoughts to have their way with you. The moment a negative thought such as, "Come on, who are you kidding? This isn't going to work," comes into your mind, catch it like a rubber ball and throw it away. Then answer it back with a counterthought: "It's a science. It has to work. The only thing that can stop it from working is if I don't do it. I'm not going to let that happen."

Negative verbalizations are just as bad as negative thinking. Every time you catch yourself verbally putting yourself down, reverse yourself. For example, if you catch yourself saying to your wife or a friend, "I'll probably never be able to keep this up," stop right there and say, "That's what I used to think. This time it's different. I can feel it in my gut."

If someone says something negative about your new commitment, don't argue with him or her. Just smile mysteriously and say, "I know what I'm doing." And in fact, it may be a good idea to keep your new workout a secret for two or three weeks, at least until you've had enough time to become hooked on the feeling and the power. Once you get that feeling, no one will be able to discourage you. In the beginning, however, you may want to protect that new seed. Keep it under the ground where the outside elements cannot damage it in its most delicate stage. Let it grow strong first. Then tell anyone you want to tell.

REMEMBER—WHEN NOTHING SEEMS TO BE HAPPENING, THE OPPOSITE IS TRUE!

Your plateau or sticking point can happen right in the beginning stages of your workout, or later on, but whenever it happens, rest assured it will happen. Why? Seeming sticking points are a part of the natural growth process. You don't see anything when you first plant a seed in the ground, do you? In fact, you have to wait weeks before you see the green seedling popping through the soil—and some seeds take longer than others to emerge. So it is with the development of the human body. You may work out for three weeks and become angry when you don't see as much progress as you had expected. Don't be discouraged. Human beings are not carbon copies of each other. Everyone has a slightly different growth process. Just keep going. Very soon the seed will pop and you will see wonderful changes. It is inevitable.

Once you start seeing improvements in your body week to week, month to month, you'll get spoiled. You'll get so used to the wonder of change that if, for a few weeks, nothing seems to be happening, you may become discouraged. You may say to yourself, "That's it. I guess this is where I stop." No. Of course it's not true. You're just experiencing a normal external hiatus—but still an internal growth time, a time when the muscles are doing something under the surface. It reminds me of how children grow. We never really see them grow, do we? In fact, when you measure a child from one year to the next, you wonder when he or she grew. You didn't see anything happening for months. Yet it happened.

It will happen. Be patient. Don't let anything shake your determination. Keep going no matter what. If you do it, I guarantee the results. You can write to me and show off your before-and-after photographs. I will personally congratulate you!

Notes:

1. Nelson Boswell, *Successful Living Day by Day* (New York: Macmillan Publishing Co., 1972), p. 130.

2. Donald Wilson, M.D., *Total Mind Power* (New York: Berkley Books, 1978), p. 12.

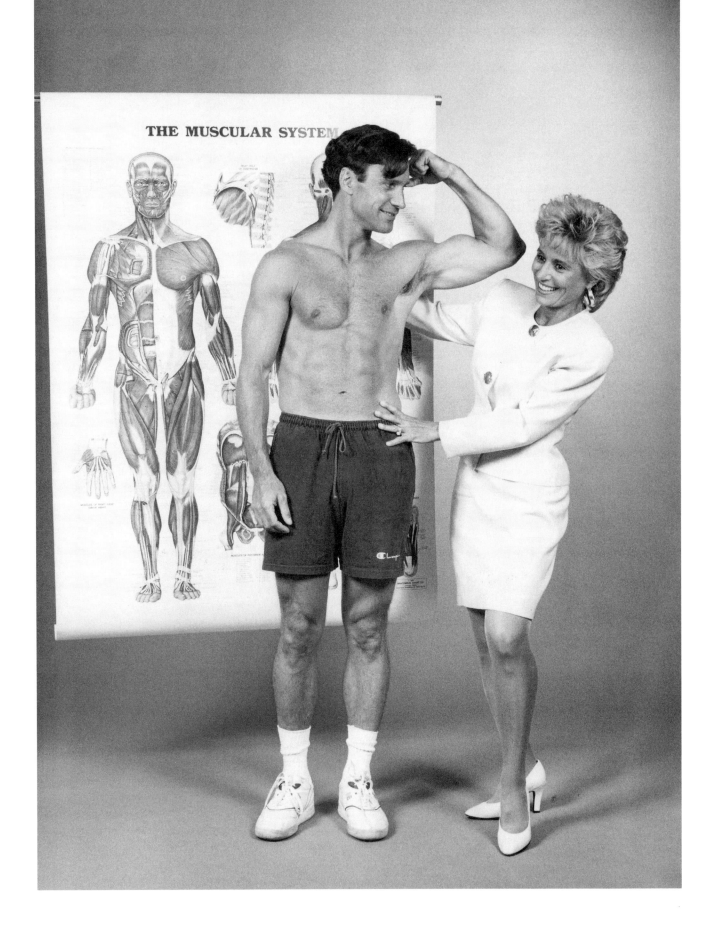

THE MUSCULAR SYSTEM

4

Fundamentals

Before you begin your workout, it's a good idea to become familiar with the terms and basic principles of the workout. Reading this chapter will not be a waste of time, because examples to demonstrate the principles are taken from the workout itself. In other words, in addition to learning the basics, you will get a preview of the workout.

The following paragraphs explain basic exercise and equipment expressions, workout principles, and terms related to muscle growth. You will also learn how to detect the difference between natural muscle soreness and injury. Finally, and perhaps most important, you will learn the function and location of the muscles involved in this workout—in the order that they appear in your workout.

BASIC EXERCISE AND EQUIPMENT TERMS

Exercise. A bodybuilding movement that is performed for a specific body part. For example, the flat dumbbell press is an exercise for the chest.

Repetition (Rep). One full movement of an exercise, from start, to midpoint, and back to start again. For example, in the flat dumbbell press, one repetition consists of raising the dumbbells from the start position of the chest-armpit area to midpoint—each arm fully extended above each pectoral (chest) muscle—and then lowering the dumbbells back to start position (the chest-armpit area).

Set. A prescribed number of repetitions. For example, in this workout, your first set of all exercises (except abdominals) will consist of twelve repetitions (reps).

Rest. A pause between sets. In this workout you will rest fifteen seconds between each set, unless you choose the giant set speed workout, or the bulk-up plan, in which case you will rest less or more (to be discussed in Chapter 5).

Breathing. The natural inhalation and exhalation of air during a workout. It is best to breathe naturally, rather than to consciously think of when to inhale and when to exhale. Powerlifters breathe out as they perform the maximum effort of the movement, due to the heaviness of the work. But most bodybuilders simply breathe naturally. The key is, do not hold your breath!

Routine. All exercises performed for a given body part. For example, your regular chest routine consists of the flat dumbbell press, the flat dumbbell flye, and the incline dumbbell press. (If you choose to do Ironman or Superman workouts, additional exercises will be added.)

Workout. All of the routines performed in a given workout session. For example, unless you choose to do the split routine, each of your workout sessions will consist of: chest, biceps, triceps, back, shoulder, and abdominal routines.

Intensity. The speed and difficulty of your workout. The more intense the workout, the more you get out of it. An example of increased intensity is increasing workout speed by decreasing or eliminating rests between sets. Increasing weights (resistance) can also increase workout intensity.

Resistance. The heaviness of the weight used in a given exercise. Since this workout is based upon the pyramid system, your first set will require your lightest resistance, your second set will require your medium resistance, and your third and final set, your heaviest resistance.

Contract. To shorten the muscle fibers by squeezing them together. For example, in this workout, when you do your seated simultaneous dumbbell curl you contract the muscle when you curl the dumbbells up toward your shoulders, shortening the muscle fibers.

Flex. To give an added, willful "squeeze" to the contracting muscle. For example, in the curl mentioned above, as you curl the dumbbell upward toward your shoulder, and as the muscle fibers contract, if you willfully squeeze the muscle as it contracts, you will have "flexed" the muscle. A way to help you flex a muscle is to imagine that a doctor were coming at your muscle with a needle, or to imagine that someone is about to punch you *hard* in that area.

Stretch. To lengthen the muscle fibers. For example, when doing the seated simultaneous dumbbell curl, you stretch your biceps muscle as you allow the dumbbells to descend to start position (your arms will have uncurled, and will be nearly straight down on either side), and the muscle fibers will have lengthened from the shortened position.

Superset. Doing a set of two different exercises without taking a rest between sets. Supersets can be done for two different exercises for the same body part, or for two different exercises for different body parts. This workout will not require supersets.

Giant Set. Doing a set of three or more different exercises without taking a rest between sets. Giant sets are usually done within one given body part. Giant sets speed up your workout, deliver greater muscle definition, and allow you to burn maximum fat (there is an aerobic effect with giant setting); but you can't work with very heavy weights because not enough time is allowed to recover and to cope with those weights. Giant setting is ideal for those people who want to burn maximum fat, save time, and build small, well-defined muscles. The giant set option will be explained in detail on pp. 58–59.

Flat Exercise Bench. A long, narrow, padded bench used to do exercises such as the flat dumbbell press.

Incline Exercise Bench. A bench that can be raised to various degrees of incline in order to perform incline exercises. For example, the incline dumbbell press is performed on an incline bench.

Bench Press Station. A device that is attached to an exercise bench consisting of bars that can hold a barbell. (Since barbells are not required for this workout, but are offered as an option, a bench press station is not required, but optional.)

Free Weights. Weights that can be carried about, as opposed to those that are permanently fixed to the ground (machines). Dumbbells, barbells, and plates are examples of free weights.

Dumbbell. A short, usually metal bar with a ball or disc attached to each end. Dumbbells can be held in each hand, as opposed to barbells, which must be held with both hands at a time.

Barbell. A long metal bar upon which weights (plates) can be placed at each end (optional).

Plates. Disc-shaped weights that can be added to either end of a barbell (optional).

Collar. A holding device placed at either end of a barbell when plates have been added, to prevent the plates from slipping off the barbell (optional).

Squat Rack. A device made to hold a barbell in the proper place so that you can step under the barbell and easily place it on your shoulders in order to do barbell squats (optional). If you want to do heavy squats, it's a good idea to use a barbell and plates, and to purchase a squat rack.

Machines. Any workout mechanism that is attached to the ground. Machines are run by air pressure, pulleys, cams, etc. Nautilus, Universal Gym, and Cybex are examples of brands of machines (optional).

FREE WEIGHTS VERSUS MACHINES

Free weights are preferred over machines by all bodybuilders because they allow you to isolate the muscle completely, and give joints and limbs the opportunity to move along their own natural planes, whereas machines force movement along specific lines dictated by the particular machine, and can put unnatural stress on the muscles.

One of the reasons people like machines so much is the machine can do most of the work if you let it. For example, you can sit in the seat of the shoulder press machine, and jerk the handle bars upward, and nearly let them drop down to place—or even completely let them drop down—and you won't get hurt. You can even fool yourself into believing that you've exercised your shoulder muscles. If you worked with dumbbells, however, you could not jerk the weights up—you would have to actually lift them—and you certainly would not be able to let them nearly drop down to your shoulders, or you would hurt yourself. You would have to control the dumbbells at all times, and of course, in the process, do all of the work.

I'm not saying that it is impossible to do all the work with a machine. It's just that it is much easier to let a machine do the work than it is to let free weights do the work!

Some machines, however, are particularly effective for exercising certain muscles, and bodybuilders regularly use them (machines are used for about one fourth of most bodybuilders' workouts). In general, these machines are the leg extension machine, the leg curl machine, the lying leg press, the lat pulldown (which can also be used for the triceps pushdown), the pulley rowing machine, the T bar row machine, and the seated and standing calf machines.

In any case, any exercise that can be done with a machine can be done with free weights. However, for those of you who own home-gym machines, or who enjoy working with machines in a gym situation, the best possible way to use the machines is described in Chapter 7.

WORKOUT PRINCIPLES

The Forty-eight-Hour Recovery Principle. The allowing of forty-eight hours (or a day of rest) before rechallenging a muscle with a weight-training workout in order to allow the muscle optimum growth and to prevent overtraining and muscle attrition. The only muscle that is an exception to this rule is the abdominal area, which can be exercised every day due to the smallness of the muscle.

Split Routine. The exercising of one half of the body on workout day one, and the other half of the body on workout day two, in order to insure maximum challenge of each body part if one is unable to do the entire workout in one day. This system allows for the individual to observe the forty-eight hour rest principle, and still work out two or more days in a row.

If you use a split routine, you never work the same body parts two days in a row (except for abdominals, which will be discussed later).

In this workout, if you choose to do the split routine, you will exercise chest, biceps, triceps, and abdominals on workout day one, and abdominals, back, shoulders, and optional thighs and calves on workout day two.

Muscle Isolation. The exercising of one muscle group completely, before advancing to the next muscle group, in order to insure maximum muscle development. For example, you would do all of your exercises for your chest (your entire chest routine) before you advanced to your next routine for that day, your biceps routine.

The Pyramid System. The adding of weight to each set of an exercise, at the expense of a few repetitions. For example, in performing your flat dumbbell press for your chest, you will do your first set of twelve repetitions, with, say, ten-pound dumbbells, your second set of ten repetitions with, say, fifteen-pound dumbbells, and your last set of six to eight repetitions, with, say, twenty-pound dumbbells. (As you get stronger, of course, you will increase your weights all the way around. This is called "progression," which will be discussed next.)

The purpose of the pyramid system is to coax the body into putting forth maximum effort without overtraining the muscle or becoming bored, and to provide a light set, which gives the muscle a natural warm-up stretch.

Technically speaking, a true pyramid would require one to go "down the pyramid" by decreasing the weights and doing more repetitions until the beginning point was reached. Over time, however, bodybuilders have come to use the true pyramid only very rarely for special contest training. They use the pyramid system as described above (sometimes called the modified pyramid system) all of the time, for all exercises except abdominals, where light or no weights are used for all sets.

Progression. The adding of weights to your overall workout, once the inital weights have become too easy to lift, and when you are tempted to increase repetitions. The purpose of progression is to force the muscles to gradually work harder and to grow or make "progress."

Cheating. Doing the last few repetitions of the last set for a given exercise in incomplete form or with assistance from the body such as a slight swing of the arms or torso because the weight is a little bit too heavy, or because an unusually short rest has been taken.

"Cheating" in this context is not really cheating, but rather a method of getting in those last few repetitions that would otherwise be lost. This kind of cheating is sometimes necessary when you have just raised your overall weights, and are not quite able to cope with the last few repetitions of the last set at the new, higher weight, or when you are getting used to the limited rests allowed when giant setting.

Priority Training. Working a difficult body part first in the workout in order to give it the first burst of energy. You may feel free to change the order of the body parts in any workout day. You may also change the order of exercises within a given body part. As long as you do all three exercises for a body part without interjecting another body part, you are following the rules.

Anaerobic Exercise. A workout that is too demanding to be supported by the body's natural oxygen supply, and so creates an oxygen deficit, forcing you to take a short rest in order to catch your breath. Although weight lifting has been traditionally considered to be an anaerobic exercise, since you will not be using extremely heavy weights in this workout you won't feel out of breath very often, and in fact will often get an aerobic effect—especially if you limit or eliminate your rests.

If you choose to do the giant set speed workout, you will work at an aerobic pace, because your rests will be few and far between, and your weights will be relatively light.

Aerobic Exercise. An exercise that can be sustained by your body's own, natural supply of oxygen, and causes your pulse to reach a rate of 60 percent to 85 percent of its capacity, and stay there for twenty minutes or longer. The Top Shape Workout has an aerobic effect, but it is even more aerobic if you choose to do the giant set speed routine.

TERMS RELATED TO MUSCLE GROWTH AND DEVELOPMENT

Mass. The size or fullness of the muscle. Notice the difference in the muscle mass in the before-and-after men. It is possible to put on about five to seven pounds of muscle mass a year, but if you are also losing fat and water weight, your scale weight will probably show up as a loss—but in the meantime, you will have gained muscle mass and changed your body composition.

Muscle as Opposed to Fat. Muscle is condensed in texture, as opposed to fat, which is airy in texture. Therefore, in terms of size, muscle weighs more than fat— or to put it a different way, muscle weighs more than fat but takes up less space. A 270 pound bodybuilder will look much thinner, and will have a much narrower waist, for example, than will a 270 pound fat man. That's why when men get in shape, they usually forget all about the scale.

Density. The hardness of the muscle. Flexing the muscle to the fullest extent while performing each repetition, decreasing rest periods, and working the muscle to capacity by using correct weights insure muscle density.

Definition. The delineation and visibility of a muscle due to lack of the presence of fat, and development of muscle density.

Muscularity. The quantity of muscle in relation to fat. The more muscle on the body in relation to fat, the more "muscularity" a person possesses.

Ripped. A muscular condition where superficial slender lines separating the muscle from other muscles can be clearly seen. A "ripped" condition is definition in the extreme, and can always be seen on champion bodybuilders as they compete in contests.

Pumped. The swelling up of the muscle beyond its normal size, due to the accelerated flow of blood through the muscle as a result of the exercise routine. The "pump" makes the exercised muscle appear larger for hours after the workout. A pump is most likely to occur when one exercises at maximum intensity and concentration.

Symmetry. The aesthetic balance and proportion of muscles in relationship to other muscles on the body. The goal of this workout is to produce the best possible symmetry for the body. In other words, it would not do to have huge biceps and underdeveloped, slumping shoulders and pectorals (chest muscles).

If you opt not to do the optional leg workout, unless you are, say, a soccer player, your lower body may not be in balance with your upper body, but you may not care about that because, like most men, chances are your legs are rarely seen in public.

Plateau or Sticking Point. A short period of time where muscles do not appear to grow or change, in spite of the fact that you are working out to full capacity. In reality, the muscle is making progress during this time; however, that progress is not visible.

Remember: Muscles grow and change the way children grow and change—they do it when no one is looking—after seeming to be making no progress.

THE DIFFERENCE BETWEEN SORENESS AND INJURY

Muscle soreness is caused by microscopic tears in the fibers of the connective tissues in your body. The slight swelling that accompanies these tears causes the soreness. When it comes to soreness in the beginning stages of your workout, unfortunately the old adage is true: "No pain, no gain." In other words, if you feel nothing at all for the first few workout sessions, you should be suspicious that nothing is happening!

Chances are some muscles will be more sore than others. You can be sure that these are your most neglected muscles. In fact, you could probably draw a "neglect" chart on your body the day after your first and second workout by marking your most sore body parts with Magic Marker. Rather than being disgusted with soreness, most men tell me that they are happy because it indicates that "something is happening."

The worst thing you could do the day you experience soreness is to not work out. Working out helps to relieve the soreness, because exercising the sore muscle forces blood to circulate through it, and in effect, massage it. If your soreness is very severe, you may use lighter weights for a day or two, but whatever you do, don't stop working out.

Soreness will go away in a few weeks—but from time to time, after a particularly challenging workout, you will feel sore again.

Injury is easy to recognize. Instead of the gradual soreness that comes the next day as a result of working out, there is a sudden and sharp, often incapacitating pain. Common injuries are fascia injuries (injuries to the material that surrounds or packages the muscle), caused by sudden jerking or pulling of the weights; tendinitis (inflammation of the tendon), caused by lifting too heavy a weight for the first set; and ligament injuries (tears or strains of the ligaments), caused by jerking the weights in an uneven manner.

If you follow the exercise instructions carefully, and perform the movements as instructed in the photographs and the directions, and if you use the pyramid system with its natural warm-up light first set, you should have no problem with injury.

If you think you might have sustained an injury, see your doctor immediately. Once you locate the problem, with your doctor's permission, you can begin working around the injury. With your doctor's permission, you may want to try *The 12-Minute Total-Body Workout* (see bibliography) as a temporary muscle-sustaining activity if you are unable to do the usual workout due to injury.

If your injury is isolated, and does not affect other body parts, your doctor may allow you to work as usual on those body parts. For example, if you have injured your leg, you may well be able to exercise your chest, shoulders, and arms in the usual manner. The key is, never stop everything unless ordered to do so by a doctor you trust.

DESCRIPTION OF MUSCLES EXERCISED IN THIS WORKOUT

Chest
(Pectoralis Major, or Pectorals, or Pecs)

The pectoral muscles are located in the upper anterior chest, and fan out, spreading from the collarbone along the breastbone and into the cartilage connecting the ribs to the breastbone. The muscle has two heads: the clavicular head of the muscle, which is the smallest of the two heads (it forms the upper pectoral area), and the larger sternal head (it forms the middle and lower pectoral area).

The pectoral muscles cooperate with the deltoid (shoulder) muscles to lift the arms and move them forward.

Biceps

This two-headed muscle is located in the front of the upper arm, between the elbow and the shoulder joint. Both heads (one is longer than the other) come together to form a "hill" about one third down the arm. The biceps functions to flex and twist the hand, and to flex the arm.

Triceps

This three-headed muscle runs along the back of the upper arm. One of the heads is attached to the shoulder blade, while the other two heads originate from the back side of the upper arm and insert at the elbow.

The longer head of the triceps muscle functions to pull the arm back once it has been moved away from the body, while the other two heads, in conjunction with the longer head, work to extend the arm and forearm.

Shoulders
(Deltoids)

The deltoid muscle gives the shoulder its shape. It is a triangular-shaped muscle that resembles an inverted version of the Greek letter delta, hence the name "deltoid." The three parts of this muscle, the anterior (front deltoid), the medial (middle and side deltoid), and the posterior (rear deltoid) can function independently, or as a group.

This muscle originates in the upper area of the shoulder blade where it joins the collarbone. The three parts of the muscle weave together and are attached on the bone of the upper arm. One angle drapes over the shoulder area, another points down the arm, weaving around the front of the arm, and the third drapes down the back of the arm.

The anterior deltoid cooperates with the pectoral muscles to lift the arm and move it forward. The medial deltoid helps to lift the arm sideways, and the posterior deltoid works in conjunction with the latissimus dorsi to extend the arm backward.

Back
(Latissimus Dorsi and Trapezius)

Although there are many muscles in the back, these are the two major muscles that we are concerned with in this workout. The latissimus dorsi muscles originate along the spinal column in the middle of the back, and travel upward and sideways to the shoulders, and insert in the front of the upper arm. These muscles give the back its greatest width, or its V shape. They function to help pull the shoulder back and downward toward the body, and to assist in pressing movements.

The trapezius is a triangular muscle that originates along the spine and runs from the back of the neck to the middle of the back. The upper fibers of the trapezius are attached to the collarbone and are evident in the shoulder area. For this reason, most people think that the "traps" are located only between the neck and shoulder area, when in reality, the muscle showing in that area is really only the tip of the iceberg.

The upper trapezius muscles function to shrug the shoulders and pull the head back, while the lower part of the muscle group helps to support the shoulder blade when the arm is raised above the head.

Abdominals
(Rectus Abdominis, External Obliques, Internal Obliques)

The abdominals or "abs" consist of one long, powerful, segmented muscle called the rectus abdominis. It functions to pull the upper body toward the lower body when sitting up from the lying-down position. The abdominals originate from the fifth through seventh rib, and run vertically up and down across the abdominal wall.

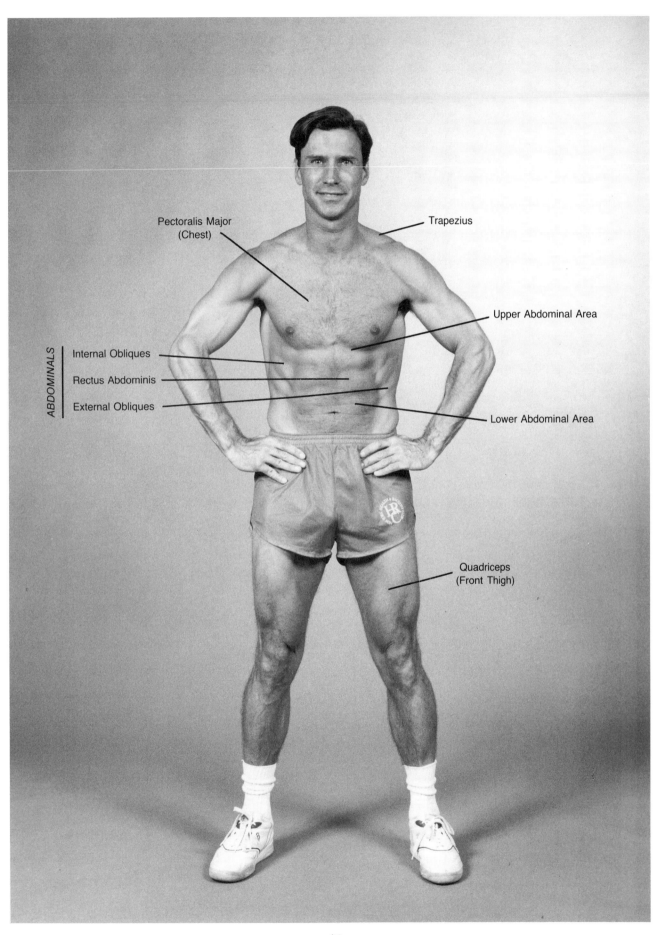

Pectoralis Major
(Chest)

Trapezius

Upper Abdominal Area

ABDOMINALS

Internal Obliques

Rectus Abdominis

External Obliques

Lower Abdominal Area

Quadriceps
(Front Thigh)

49

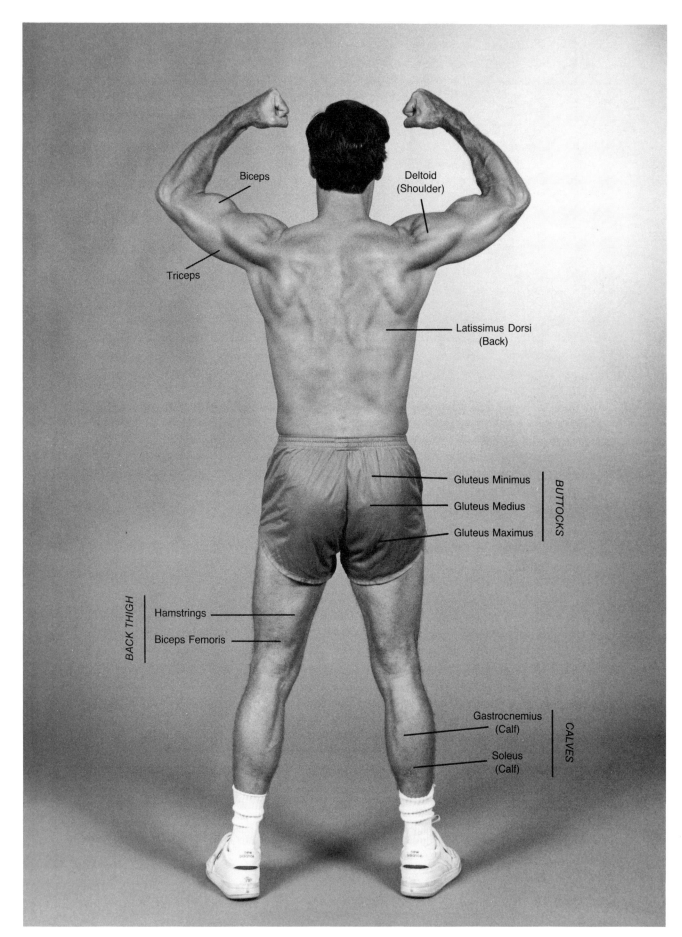

Biceps

Deltoid
(Shoulder)

Triceps

Latissimus Dorsi
(Back)

Gluteus Minimus

Gluteus Medius

Gluteus Maximus

BUTTOCKS

BACK THIGH

Hamstrings

Biceps Femoris

Gastrocnemius
(Calf)

Soleus
(Calf)

CALVES

Although the rectus abdominis is actually one long, segmented muscle, abdominals are exercised in sections: upper and lower, because it is difficult to challenge the entire muscle sufficiently with one exercise.

The external oblique muscles originate at the side of the lower ribs and run diagonally to the rectus abdominis. They are attached to the sheath of fibrous tissue that surrounds the rectus abdominis. These muscles function with other muscles to rotate and flex the torso.

The internal oblique muscles run at right angles to the external oblique muscles. It is this angle that determines the width of the waistline. The greater the slant of the oblique muscles, the smaller the waist. The exercises that challenge the external and internal oblique muscles help to remove the notorious love handles. These exercises also help to form diagonal lines of definition in the side-abdominal area that help to make the waist appear smaller.

Front and Back Thigh
(Quadriceps and Hamstrings)

The front thigh or quadriceps is a group of four muscles: the rectus femoris and three vasti muscles. The rectus femoris originates on a ridge on the front of the hip bone, while the three vasti muscles originate in various parts of the thigh bone. The four muscles are joined at the kneecap. The quadriceps muscle group works to extend the leg from the bent-knee position.

The back thigh is composed of the biceps femoris and semimembranosus and semitendinosus muscles. Together this group of muscles is called the hamstrings.

The biceps femoris is a two-headed muscle that works in cooperation with the semimembranosus and semitendinosus muscles to flex the knee, rotate the leg, and extend the hips. These muscles originate in the bony area of the pelvis and end along the back knee joint.

Calf
(Gastrocnemius and Soleus)

The gastrocnemius is a two-headed muscle that connects in the middle of the lower leg and ties in with the Achilles tendon. The point where the two muscles are connected forms the calf muscle. This muscle helps to bend the knee and flex the foot downward. It works in opposition to the extensor muscles of the lower leg, which pull the foot downward.

The soleus muscle originates on the back of the tibia and the head of the fibula bones. It lies underneath the gastrocnemius muscle, but does not pass the knee joint. For this reason, it functions only to flex the foot downward, but cannot help to bend the knee.

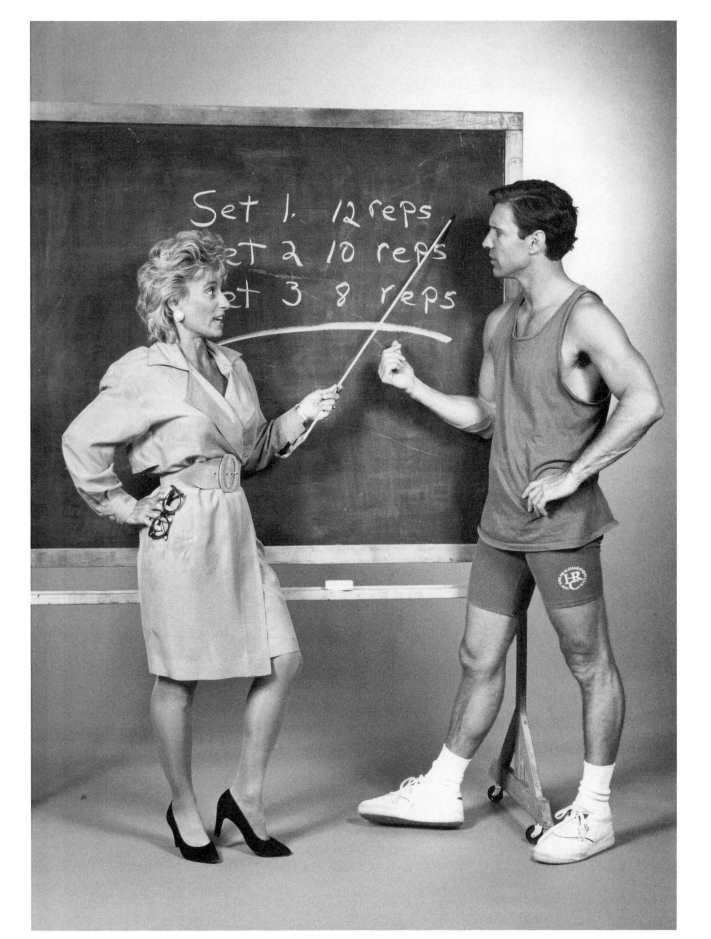

5

How to Do the Workout

This chapter will tell you exactly how to do the Top Shape Workout, and how to advance to the Ironman and Superman workouts if you so desire. It will explain the difference between the forty-minute, three-day-a-week plan, and the thirty-minute, four-day-a-week split routine, and give options to work with weights up to six days a week. It will also explain how to set up a workout schedule, and how to incorporate aerobics into your routine if you have the time.

For those of you who want to speed up your workout—making it only twenty minutes, and at the same time burn maximum fat, but get smaller, more defined muscles—the giant set speed workout will be explained; and for those of you who want to build bigger muscles than the regular program allows, or to "bomb" certain lagging body parts, special instructions are given.

Finally, home and gym workout options are discussed, and a break-in-gently plan is presented. In short, by the time you finish reading this chapter, you'll know everything you need to know—and you'll be ready to start your workout.

THE FORTY-MINUTE, THREE-DAY-A-WEEK PLAN: SETS, REPETITIONS, AND WEIGHTS

You will do three sets for each exercise—no matter what exercise you are doing—and you will add weight to each set at the expense of a few repetitions (the pyramid system; see pp. 4 and 43 for a review of this principle). You will do this for every exercise except abdominal exercises, which require no weight or a light dumbbell. This exception will be discussed later in the chapter.

Note: When the term "dumbbells" is used, the weight mentioned refers to *each* dumbbell. For example, "ten-pound dumbbells" means that each dumbbell weighs ten pounds.

Here is the workout.

CHEST ROUTINE

Flat Dumbbell Press

Set 1:	12 reps	10-pound dumbbells	(Rest 15 seconds)
Set 2:	10 reps	15-pound dumbbells	(Rest 15 seconds)
Set 3:	6 to 8 reps	20-pound dumbbells	(Rest 15 seconds)

Flat Dumbbell Flye

Set 1:	12 reps	10-pound dumbbells	(Rest 15 seconds)
Set 2:	10 reps	15-pound dumbbells	(Rest 15 seconds)
Set 3:	6 to 8 reps	20-pound dumbbells	(Rest 15 seconds)

Incline Dumbbell Press

Set 1:	12 reps	10-pound dumbbells	(Rest 15 seconds)
Set 2:	10 reps	15-pound dumbbells	(Rest 15 seconds)
Set 3:	6 to 8 reps	20-pound dumbbells	

You rest the same 15 seconds and begin your

BICEPS ROUTINE

Seated Simultaneous Dumbbell Curl with a Twist

Set 1:	12 reps	10-pound dumbbells	(Rest 15 seconds)
Set 2:	10 reps	15-pound dumbbells	(Rest 15 seconds)
Set 3:	6 to 8 reps	20-pound dumbbells	(Rest 15 seconds)

Seated Alternate Hammer Curl

Set 1:	12 reps	10-pound dumbbells	(Rest 15 seconds)
Set 2:	10 reps	15-pound dumbbells	(Rest 15 seconds)
Set 3:	6 to 8 reps	20-pound dumbbells	(Rest 15 seconds)

Concentration Curl with a Twist

Set 1:	12 reps	10-pound dumbbells	(Rest 15 seconds)
Set 2:	10 reps	15-pound dumbbells	(Rest 15 seconds)
Set 3:	6 to 8 reps	20-pound dumbbells	

You rest the same 15 seconds and begin your

TRICEPS ROUTINE

Lying Dumbbell Exension

Set 1:	12 reps	10-pound dumbbells	(Rest 15 seconds)
Set 2:	10 reps	15-pound dumbbells	(Rest 15 seconds)
Set 3:	6 to 8 reps	20-pound dumbbells	(Rest 15 seconds)

One-Arm Triceps Kickback with a Twist

Set 1:	12 reps	10-pound dumbbells	(Rest 15 seconds)
Set 2:	10 reps	15-pound dumbbells	(Rest 15 seconds)
Set 3:	6 to 8 reps	20-pound dumbbells	(Rest 15 seconds)

Seated One-Arm Triceps Overhead Extension with a Twist

Set 1:	12 reps	10-pound dumbbells	(Rest 15 seconds)
Set 2:	10 reps	15-pound dumbbells	(Rest 15 seconds)
Set 3:	6 to 8 reps	20-pound dumbbells	

You rest the same 15 seconds and begin your

ABDOMINAL ROUTINE

Alternate Knee-in

Set 1:	12 reps	10-pound dumbbells	(Rest 15 seconds)
Set 2:	10 reps	15-pound dumbbells	(Rest 15 seconds)
Set 3:	6 to 8 reps	20-pound dumbbells	(Rest 15 seconds)

Knee-Raised Crunch

Set 1:	12 reps	10-pound dumbbells	(Rest 15 seconds)
Set 2:	10 reps	15-pound dumbbells	(Rest 15 seconds)
Set 3:	6 to 8 reps	20-pound dumbbells	(Rest 15 seconds)

Squatting Side Bend

Set 1:	12 reps	10-pound dumbbells	(Rest 15 seconds)
Set 2:	10 reps	15-pound dumbbells	(Rest 15 seconds)
Set 3:	6 to 8 reps	20-pound dumbbells	

You rest the same 15 seconds and begin your

BACK ROUTINE

Double-Arm Bent Dumbbell Row

Set 1:	12 reps	10-pound dumbbells	(Rest 15 seconds)
Set 2:	10 reps	15-pound dumbbells	(Rest 15 seconds)
Set 3:	6 to 8 reps	20-pound dumbbells	(Rest 15 seconds)

Single-Arm Bent Dumbbell Row

Set 1:	12 reps	10-pound dumbbells	(Rest 15 seconds)
Set 2:	10 reps	15-pound dumbbells	(Rest 15 seconds)
Set 3:	6 to 8 reps	20-pound dumbbells	(Rest 15 seconds)

Upright Row

Set 1:	12 reps	10-pound dumbbells	(Rest 15 seconds)
Set 2:	10 reps	15-pound dumbbells	(Rest 15 seconds)
Set 3:	6 to 8 reps	20-pound dumbbells	

You rest the same 15 seconds and begin your final routine

SHOULDER ROUTINE

Seated Simultaneous Dumbbell Press

Set 1:	12 reps	10-pound dumbbells	(Rest 15 seconds)
Set 2:	10 reps	15-pound dumbbells	(Rest 15 seconds)
Set 3:	6 to 8 reps	20-pound dumbbells	(Rest 15 seconds)

Seated Side Lateral

Set 1:	12 reps	10-pound dumbbells	(Rest 15 seconds)
Set 2:	10 reps	15-pound dumbbells	(Rest 15 seconds)
Set 3:	6 to 8 reps	20-pound dumbbells	(Rest 15 seconds)

Standing Bent Lateral with a Twist

Set 1:	12 reps	10-pound dumbbells	(Rest 15 seconds)
Set 2:	10 reps	15-pound dumbbells	(Rest 15 seconds)
Set 3:	6 to 8 reps	20-pound dumbbells	

You have exercised the following body parts:

chest
biceps
triceps
abdominals
back
shoulders

You will do the workout on any three days of the week. The only requirement is that you leave one day off between workouts. For example, you can work out on Monday, Wednesday, Friday; Tuesday, Thursday, Saturday; Sunday, Tuesday, Thursday; and so on. If you wish to do aerobics on your days off, that is fine, but if you want to work with weights two or more days in a row, you will have to switch to a split routine. Reasons for this are explained on pp. 5 and 43. Suggested workout plans are discussed later in this chapter.

IRONMAN AND SUPERMAN ROUTINES

If you wish to perfect your body even further, you can go the extra mile and add one or two exercises to each body part. If you do, you proceed with the workout exactly as above, only you will add the exercises given at the end of each exercise chapter. If you do the Ironman workout, you will be doing four exercises per body part instead of the usual three. If you choose to do the Superman workout, you will be doing five exercises per body part.

What if you want to do Ironman or Superman only for certain body parts? No problem. For example, say you want to do extra work for your shoulders, but you are happy with your biceps with just the three exercises. Simply add the exercises for your shoulders only. It's up to you to decide where you need the extra work.

If you do all of the Ironman additions, you will add ten minutes to your total workout time, bringing your workout up to fifty minutes. If you do the Superman routine, you will add yet another ten minutes to your total workout time, bringing your workout up to a full hour. Since this is a long workout, you may decide that you would like to do a split routine, but if you have the energy, more power to you. You can do it all in one day, unless of course you choose to do the leg option. That would be too much work for one day. (See pp. 132–144.)

SMALLER, MORE DEFINED MUSCLES AND SHORTER WORKOUTS: THE GIANT SET SPEED PLAN WORKOUT

The giant set requires that you do your first set of three or more exercises before you take a rest. Let's use the chest routine as an example. It consists of:

Flat Dumbbell Press
Flat Dumbbell Flye
Incline Dumbbell Press

Here's how it works. You do your first set of the flat dumbbell press of twelve repetitions and, without resting, you do your first set of twelve repetitions of the flat dumbbell flye, and again, without resting, you do your first set of the twelve repetitions of the incline dumbbell press. You will, of course, have used your first weight, the ten-pound dumbbells.

Now you take a big fifteen-second rest.

Then you do your second set of ten repetitions of the flat dumbbell press, and, without resting, you do your second set of ten repetitions of the flat dumbbell flye, and again, without resting, you do your second set of ten repetitions of the incline dumbbell press. Of course, you will have used your second weight, the fifteen-pound dumbbells.

Now you rest a big fifteen seconds.

Then you do your third and last giant set, of six to eight repetitions of the flat dumbbell press, the flat dumbbell flye, and the incline dumbbell press. You will have of course used your heaviest weight, your twenty-pound dumbbells.

You will then take a big fifteen-second rest and immediately move to your biceps routine, and so on, until you have completed all six body parts—your entire workout. You can see where you will have shaved off ten minutes from the routine by having eliminated more than half of the rests! The entire workout will take you twenty minutes.

Besides saving time, you get the bonus of maximum fat burning because you keep your heart within the ideal fat-burning range of 60 percent to 70 percent of capacity. However, if your goal is to significantly increase your muscle size, you should not use this workout, because you are not resting long enough between sets in order to let the muscles recuperate sufficiently to use heavy-enough weights. In fact, although I explained the routine with the regular ten-, fifteen-, and twenty-pound dumbbells, the truth is, you will have to start out with eight-, ten-, and twelve-pound dumbbells and build up to the tens, fifteens, and twenties in time!

Note that if you were doing the Ironman or Superman workouts, you would have added one or two exercises to each giant set, making the complete giant set four or five sets of four or five different exercises without a rest!

If you have any doubt that the giant set speed method works, consult the half a million people who bought and used my best-selling book, *The Fat-Burning Workout*. It is exactly the method used in that book!

THE THIRTY-MINUTE, FOUR-DAY-A-WEEK PLAN: THE SPLIT ROUTINE

Why do a split routine? First, you might not want to work out as long as forty minutes per session. Second, you may have chosen to add Ironman or Superman workouts to your routine, and you may not feel like working out for fifty minutes to an hour per session. Third, and most important, you may want to take advantage of the leg workout option. If you do, you must do the split routine, because trying to work eight body parts in one workout session is too much. By the end of the workout you will lose your concentration and cheat your last body parts.

You do the split routine workout exactly as above, except that you break the workout up into two parts.

WORKOUT DAYS ONE AND THREE	WORKOUT DAYS TWO AND FOUR
chest	abdominals
biceps	back
triceps	shoulders
abdominals	thighs (optional)
	calves (optional)

Notice that abdominals are repeated. Why? They must be exercised at least three to four times a week. If you have chosen the regular routine, you will exercise them three days a week. If you have chosen the split routine, all the better, you will exercise them four days a week. In fact, if you have the time, and you want to speed up your abdominal progress, you can work them as much as six times a week! (For even more abdominal options, see my book *Gut Busters*.)

The big key to the split routine is, except for abdominals, you never exercise the same muscles on two training days in a row. In other words, whatever body parts you exercised the last time you worked out, you do not exercise the next time you work out. It's that simple.

But believe it or not, you may forget from one workout to the next, so it's a good idea to mark it down on a calendar, otherwise in the middle of your workout you may realize that you exercised these body parts the last time, and have to stop and start all over with the correct body parts. (Of course, if you were using the three-day plan, this could never happen, because you would be doing the same thing every time you worked out.)

By way of reminder, the reason for the split routine, and for the day of rest betwen workouts if you don't use the split routine, is the forty-eight-hour rest principle that must not be violated. (See pp. 4 and 43 for a review of this principle.)

WHAT IF YOU WANT TO WORK WITH WEIGHTS MORE THAN FOUR DAYS A WEEK?

The same rule applies. You can do it, but you must use the split routine, meaning you never exercise the same body parts you exercised the last time you worked out. The beauty of the system is, you can work out with weights six days in a row without violating the forty-eight-hour rest principle.

Why not work with weights seven days a week? Not a good idea, because you will eventually become mentally and physically burned out. Believe me, if they could get away with working out seven days a week, bodybuilders would do it in a minute. But they don't. Even champion bodybuilders take one day off a week. I guess they took their cue from a higher source. After all, even God rested on the seventh day!

SOME MUSCLES ARE WEAKER THAN OTHERS

For the sake of simplicity, I recommend the use of ten-, fifteen-, and twenty-pound dumbbells for all body parts, but chances are you will have to go much lighter in the beginning for the weaker muscles: triceps and shoulders, for example.

In fact, it's a good idea to use five-, eight-, and ten-pound dumbbells for these body parts in the beginning, and gradually build up to the higher weights in time. If you don't want to purchase these lighter weights, you can simply use the ten-pound dumbbells for all three sets, until you get strong enough to pyramid the weights.

WHAT IF YOU CAN'T GET THE MINIMUM NUMBER OF REPETITIONS WITH THE WEIGHT YOU ARE USING?

The answer is simple: either go lighter, or do as many repetitions with that weight as you can until you get strong enough to do the required number. For example, say you don't want to purchase lighter weights, but you can only get eight repetitions with the ten-pound dumbbells for your first set of your shoulder exercises, when you should be getting twelve repetitions, and you can only get seven repetitions for your second set with that same light weight, when you should be getting ten repetitions with a higher weight, and only four or five repetitions for your last set with that light weight, when you should be getting six to eight with a higher weight. Fine. Use the ten-pound dumbbells for a week or two, until you get stronger and find yourself doing twelve repetitions for your first set. Then and only then, start using your fifteen-pound dumbbells for your second set. At that point you may find that you can only get seven of the required ten repetitions with the fifteen-pound dumbbells for your second set, and five of the six to eight required repetitions for your last set. Use the fifteens for your second and third sets until you are getting the full required ten repetitions with the fifteen-pound dumbbells for your second set. Then add your twenty pounds for your last set. Even if you only get four of the required six to eight repetitions for that last set at first, don't worry. In a few weeks you will be getting six to eight reps with the twenty-pound dumbbells. Everything in time.

WHEN THE WEIGHTS BECOME TOO EASY TO LIFT— DO NOT INCREASE YOUR REPS, INCREASE YOUR WEIGHTS

"I'm up to twenty repetitions on my bench press," bragged one of the before-and-after men, thinking that I would praise him. "I'll kill you," I exclaimed in horror. "I thought I told you not to go over twelve repetitions—didn't I clearly explain that if the weights became too easy, you should raise your weights, not increase your repetitions? That's the whole point of the principle of progression!" "I know," he said sheepishly, "but I thought . . ."

Gentlemen, when it comes to this workout, don't think so much. Don't be creative. In fact, be a robot. Follow the workout exactly. There is no other way I can guarantee the results. Please. Trust me. Later, when you know what you're doing you can do whatever you want (after I see your before-and-after photograph). For now, rest assured, anything that you add or change will be wrong. Don't do it.

So what should you do if you find that you can do more repetitions with the weights you are using? Simple. Raise your weights all the way around. This, in fact, is exactly what the principle of progression is all about—raising your weights when the weights you are lifting become too easy, so that your muscles make progress, and become thicker, stronger, better shaped, and more defined. (See p. 43 for a review of the principle of progression.)

So if the weights become too easy (as well they will in a few weeks or a month), raise them. If you do fifty repetitions for your chest, you may be as proud as a peacock, but you will have nothing to show for it but a sunken chest.

But how heavy will the weights eventually get, and how often will you have to raise them? Chances are you will raise your weights in about three weeks, and then after two or three weeks, and then again in a month or two. Then you'll reach a plateau and leave your weights as they are. You may end up with twenty-, twenty-five-, and thirty-pound dumbbells or slightly higher. If you choose to do the giant set speed workout, however, you may remain at ten, fifteen, and twenty because it is difficult to handle much more weight when you are moving that fast; but remember, that system promises smaller muscles in the first place.

STAYING AT THE SAME WEIGHT WHEN YOU REACH A PLATEAU AND ARE HAPPY WITH YOUR SIZE

Everyone reaches a plateau of weights after a while—a comfort zone where he or she can remain forever. If you do this, you will simply stop growing bigger muscles. You will probably reach a plateau after four or five months. If you are happy with your muscle size at that point, don't continue to push yourself to lift heavier and heavier. Remain there. You will maintain that size and continue to gain in hardness and definition.

BOMBING TECHNIQUES

After you have been working out for *at least three months* (you may want to wait six months, just to be sure your body part doesn't catch up on its own), and your body is basically transformed, you may notice that certain body parts are lagging behind. If this is the case, you may want to employ special "bombing techniques" to those body parts. Here are some suggestions.

Muscle Priority Training

Train the lagging body part first. In other words, if your back is lagging behind your other body parts, and you are on the three-day routine, which would require you to exercise your back next to last in your routine, instead, exercise it first, giving it your first shot of energy. By giving your troublesome body part your first attention, you will be training that area harder, and it should make a difference.

Go Heavier by "Cheating"

If you have a body part that is lagging behind other body parts in size because you are too weak to lift the heavier weights that would be necessary in order to significantly increase its size, try the "cheating" method. This is one case where cheating is allowed. Here's how it works.

You can sacrifice strictness of form for the last few repetitions of a set in order to do that set with heavier weights. For example, if your shoulders are lagging behind, and you have been unable to raise your overall weights very much because, in order to do so, you would have to sacrifice strictness of form for the last few reps of each set, raise your weights anyway.

Suppose you are performing your seated simultaneous dumbbell press. Instead of following the Tips section that warns you not to jerk the dumbbells up for the last few repetitions of your set, in order to go heavier, jerk the dumbbells up! By employing this method, eventually you will get stronger, and your muscles will get bigger and be reshaped, and you will be able to go even heavier. You will continue to employ cheating methods until your underdeveloped body part catches up with the rest of your body.

Burns

The burn method involves a different form of cheating—the stealing of a few extra repetitions at the end of the last set of a given exercise. For example, if your chest is underdeveloped, and you are performing the flat dumbbell press, after you have performed your first set of twelve repetitions, and your second set of ten repetitions, and your last set of six to eight repetitions, "cheat out" a few more reps, even if you have to do half reps.

In the case of the incline dumbbell press, it may mean pushing the dumbbells up only half or three quarters of the way for each repetition. Get as many as you can until you feel a "burn" in your pectoral (chest) muscles.

The reason for saving the burn method for your last set of the exercise is obvious: if you tried it for your first set, it would backfire, and you wouldn't be able to perform as many repetitions for your next set!

Use the Extra Exercises in the Ironman and Superman Workouts

Do one (as found in the Ironman workout) or two (as found in the Superman workout) extra exercises for that body part (if you are not already using those routines). The extra exercises will insure that your lagging muscle is being attacked from additional angles, and will help to shape and develop that muscle to its optimum form.

Use the Alternatives

Attack the body part from yet other angles by periodically taking advantage of the alternatives. This may involve purchasing a barbell and some plates, but it will be worth it in the long run.

Add One Set to Each Exercise of the Routine

For example, if your biceps are lagging behind, you would add one set to each of your biceps exercises. This would change your repetitions for each set as well as your weights. Let's look at the first biceps exercise.

Seated Simultaneous Dumbbell Curl with a Twist

Set 1:	15 reps	10 pounds
Set 2:	12 reps	15 pounds
Set 3:	10 reps	20 pounds
Set 4:	6 to 8 reps	25 pounds

WHAT IF YOU WANT TO PUT ON SIGNIFICANT SIZE IN GENERAL?

If you want to put on significant size, you will have to increase your weights—but in order to do this, you will have to rest longer between sets. For example, if you rested thirty seconds between sets instead of fifteen seconds, you could handle slightly heavier weights, and if you rested forty-five seconds between sets, you could lift even heavier weights. If you rested a full minute, you could go even heavier.

If you do want to put on significant size, however, don't try to do it right away. Use the regular workout for at least three or four months. Then go into the size-building method. It's better to give your body a good chance to get used to working out before demanding that it go heavy.

ABDOMINALS CAN BE TRAINED UP TO SIX DAYS A WEEK, REQUIRE FIFTEEN TO TWENTY-FIVE REPETITIONS PER SET, AND ARE EXERCISED WITH LITTLE OR NO WEIGHT

The abdominal muscles are small and do not require much building; therefore, they can be trained often (you will not overtrain them or wear them down), need high repetitions per set, and are exercised with little or no weight.

As mentioned above, you must exercise your abdominal muscles a minimum of three days a week, and, if you want to make fast progress, you can work them up to six times a week.

What has not been mentioned so far is repetitions. You must do fifteen to twenty-five repetitions for every set of abdominal exercises—without weight. (Later, you can place a ten-, fifteen-, or twenty-pound dumbbell on your stomach, or a ten-pound dumbbell between your feet for certain exercises. See individual instructions in exercise chapters.)

If you can't get fifteen repetitions per set in the beginning, don't worry. Just do as many repetitions as you can per set. You can add one more repetition each time you work out, until you are up the full fifteen to twenty-five. Even if it takes two months to get up to the full range, don't worry. You will get there. Muscles need time and patience. Don't for one moment dream that you will never get there. It's not true. Men who were only able to do two or three reps in the beginning find themselves breezing through the program of fifteen to twenty-five reps in a matter of months.

CHANGING THE ORDER OF THE BODY PARTS

There is nothing sacred about the given order of the body parts in a workout day. As mentioned above, it is always a good idea to exercise your weakest body part first. On the other hand, you may want to change the order of body parts for a different reason.

For example, you may be the type of guy who hates to exercise abdominals, and you know that if you don't do that body part first, you will be tempted to skip it. If this is the case, you may want to exercise abdominals first. On the other hand, you may be the type who needs to exercise a "fun" body part first. If this is the case, pick your favorite body part and do it first.

CHANGING THE ORDER OF THE EXERCISES WITHIN A GIVEN BODY PART

There is also nothing sacred about the order of the exercises within a given body part. The exercises have been placed in that order for positioning purposes—so that you will not have to jump back and forth from one position to another—where possible. If, for any reason, however, you want to change the order of exercises within a body part, feel free to do it, but don't you dare start to jump around wildly from one body part to another. For example, if you are doing your chest routine, I don't care which of your chest exercises you do first, second, third, and so on, but don't do an exercise for another body part until you've done all of your chest exercises!

THE AEROBIC OPTION

Aerobics are excellent for conditioning your heart and lungs, and for burning additional body fat. In addition, aerobics will help you to do this workout without getting out of breath. So if you are already doing an aerobic activity, by all means continue to do so, and if you are not, consider adding them into your routine. Running on the treadmill, riding the stationary bicycle, or riding a regular bicycle, using a stair-stepper, jumping rope, swimming, or some such thing, for twenty to thirty mintues three to six times a week, in addition to this workout, would be the ideal combination.

But the fact is, if you only have time to do one thing, put your time into the weights, because not only will weights reshape your body by increasing and defining muscle, but they will increase bone density, make you stronger, improve your sport, and in addition, give you somewhat of an aerobic effect—especially if you do the giant set speed routine.

MAKING A SCHEDULE

If you are doing the three-day routine, your schedule may look like this ("Weights" mean the Top Shape Workout):

Sunday	Monday	Tuesday	Wednesday	Thursday	Friday	Saturday
	Weights		Weights		Weights	

If you are doing the three-day-a-week routine, and you want to fit aerobics into your schedule, here is how it may look:

Sunday	Monday	Tuesday	Wednesday	Thursday	Friday	Saturday
Aerobics	Weights		Weights	Aerobics	Weights	Aerobics

Or, you might be the type of guy who likes to get it all over with in one day. If so, your schedule may look like this:

Sunday	Monday	Tuesday	Wednesday	Thursday	Friday	Saturday
	Weights		Aerobics		Weights	
	Aerobics		Weights		Aerobics	

If you are going to do both in one workout session, which should you do first, aerobics or weights? I would do weights first because I'd like to make sure I have my full strength for those exercises. However, you can experiment. Some men find the aerobics to be a stimulating warm-up for the weight workout.

If you are on a four-day split routine your schedule may look like this:

Sunday	Monday	Tuesday	Wednesday	Thursday	Friday	Saturday
	Weights	Weights		Weights	Weights	

You can even work out with weights four days in a row, if that's best for your schedule. Since you are on a split routine, your muscles will not suffer. Of course if you have the opportunity, it's always ideal to spread your workout out over time. Why let the muscles lie stagnant for three days if you don't have to do it? Balance is always the ideal. But the beauty of the split routine is, if your schedule demands it, you can work out four days in a row.

If you are on a four-day split routine and you want to do aerobics, your schedule may look something like this:

Sunday	Monday	Tuesday	Wednesday	Thursday	Friday	Saturday
Aerobics	Weights	Weights	Aerobics	Weights	Weights	Aerobics

67

And if you want to work with weights six days a week and do aerobics six days a week, nothing is stopping you. Your schedule can look like this:

Sunday	Monday	Tuesday	Wednesday	Thursday	Friday	Saturday
Aerobics	Weights	Weights	Weights	Weights	Weights	Weights
	Aerobics	Aerobics	Aerobics	Aerobics		Aerobics

Notice that you have taken one day off a week from aerobics and one day off a week from weights. No matter how fanatical you are, you must do that or you may wear your muscles down and/or eventually experience burnout. In addition, you will increase your chance for injury because you deny the body a chance to recuperate.

THE GYM OR THE HOME—WHICH IS BETTER?

Some men would never work out at home. The very idea of working alone turns them off. They would rather go to a fitness center where other men are working out, and where they can take advantage of the energetic atmosphere and enjoy male camaraderie. They also enjoy the encouragement other men give them when they see the progress being made. A nod, a look, a compliment, and even competition can be inspirational.

On the other hand, in the gym, there are temptations and distractions. Time can be wasted in conversations between sets, causing you to take much longer than a fifteen-second rest, and decreasing the intensity and efficacy of your workout. (If you think men don't shmooze in the gym, do a little eavesdropping. You'd be amazed. They talk about everything from sports to politics to women! I know. I've heard them.)

Another thing to avoid in a gym is endless comparisons of your body with the bodies of other men. Some men who go to the gym spend more time agonizing over the shape of their bodies in relationship to other men than they do on their workout. If you go to a gym, remember, the idea is to focus your mind on your working muscle, and to use visualization as to how your body will look, not to put yourself down or to feel competitive with other men who have a whole different set of genetics. Forget about the other men. Look at yourself. It's your time to grow. All the looking in the world won't put an ounce of muscle on your body.

Another obvious disadvantage of a gym is travel time. You could have completed at least two workouts in the time it takes most people to get to and from the gym, not to mention the time it takes to dress and undress, shower, etc. So if time is of the essence, a home workout wins hands down.

Then there's the psychological part. The very thought of traveling to a gym is enough to make some men quit before they start. Such men are much happier going home and heading straight to the weights and the bench, and getting it over with in thirty or forty minutes.

Finally there's the money. It costs a lot less than a year's gym membership to purchase a bench and a few sets of dumbbells that will last you a lifetime.

CHOOSING A GYM

If you are planning to do the workout in a gym, the most important thing to consider is the availability of free weights. Ironically, the most expensive equipment, machines of every sort, are always in abundance in virtually all fitness centers, but too often free weights are not.

Make sure there are at least sets (preferably double sets, so that you will not have to wait if they are in use) of ten-, fifteen-, and twenty-pound dumbbells, and ideally also a few sets of lower weights and a few sets of higher weights. This way, if you want to begin with lower weights for your weaker body parts, you can do it, and when you are ready to advance to higher weights, they are there for you.

As far as juice bars, thick rugs, plush locker rooms, swimming pools, steam rooms, and saunas, the choice is yours. As long as you determine to ignore all distractions until you finish your workout, any gym will do. But I must admit, sometimes it is easier to work out in the least elaborate gym, because that is often where you will find bodybuilders who are there for one reason, and one reason alone—to shape their body into its most perfect form, and bodybuilders, you can be sure, are not going to try to engage you in conversation. But they will be able to give you an accurate answer to a question you might have about an exercise— if you don't interrupt them in the middle of a set.

PURCHASING YOUR DUMBBELLS AND BENCH

You can purchase inexpensive dumbbells, and a bench that goes to an incline, at any store that sells hard-core gym equipment, or at most sporting goods stores, or, if you're too busy to go shopping, and you don't mind paying the shipping charges, you can order them from me (see p. 240).

PERSONAL TRAINERS

You don't need a personal trainer with this workout. The photographs and exercise instructions are your personal trainer. However, if you do have a personal trainer, ask him or her to go through this workout with you. You will not need him or her for more than three sessions.

I, in fact, am constantly asked to do personal training. I've done it a few times, and lo and behold, I put myself out of business after three sessions. Why? People who do this workout do the real thing. They get the results once they are on the full program. The last thing they need is someone to lean on. Unfortunately, too often personal trainers function as just that—crutches for people who are afraid to stand alone.

If you do get a personal trainer, and I cannot emphasize this enough, refuse to let him or her change anything in the workout. I simply cannot guarantee the results if you allow that. If he or she is willing to follow the workout exactly, great. A personal trainer cannot hurt—but again, you won't need one for very long.

A HOME-GYM MACHINE—IF YOU HAVE THE SPACE
AND THE MONEY

A nice luxury to have is a complete home gym—so that you can add the key exercises that bodybuilders do on machines—the lat pulldown, the pulley row, the triceps pushdown, the leg extension, and a few more. In addition, there are some exercises that you can do on the machine for variety's sake. So if you have the space, and if you can afford it, by all means, purchase a home gym. But realize that the crucial part of your workout is the dumbbells and a simple bench that goes to an incline. The home-gym machine is a luxury. (See Chapter 7 for the machine workout.)

BREAKING IN GENTLY

If you go full force into the workout from day one, unless you have already been doing a very similar workout, you can be sure that the next day practically every muscle in your body will be crying out with soreness. This may discourage you and cause you to be tempted to quit the workout, so it's a much better idea to invest a few weeks, if necessary, to breaking in gently.

I must admit, though, that only one of the before-and-after men in Chapter 2 followed my advice. The others went full force into the routine and experienced incredible soreness the next day. Amazingly, they seemed to like it—even though they complained.

BREAKING IN IF YOU HAVE ALREADY BEEN WORKING
WITH WEIGHTS

If you have recently been following a workout such as the ones found in any of my fitness books, *Now or Never, The Fat-Burning Workout, Bottoms Up!,* or even *The 12 Minute Total-Body Workout,* or any bodybuilding routine that requires at least six sets of exercises per body part, you can go full force into the routine from day one—only take longer rests between sets, and feel out whether or not you should pyramid the weights, or use the ten-pound dumbbells for all three sets.

For example, you may want to use the ten-pound dumbbells for all three sets for your first workout, and add the fifteen-pound dumbbells for your second and third sets for your second workout, and then, for your third workout, add in the twenty-pound dumbbells. By the end of one week, you will be doing the full workout with all three weights—using the pyramid system.

Even though you are used to working with weights, you may still be sore the next day. Why? You will have exercised the muscles from a different angle (each new exercise hits the muscle at a slightly different angle). Be happy if you are sore. It's a sure sign that you are making progress.

BREAKING IN IF YOU HAVE LITTLE OR NO EXPERIENCE IN WORKING WITH WEIGHTS

Week 1.   Do the first set *only* of each exercise (you do twelve repetitions with your ten-pound dumbbells for this set).

Week 2.   Do your first and second set of each exercise. You will do your first set as above, rest fifteen seconds, and do ten repetitions with your fifteen-pound dumbbell for your second set.

Week 3.   Do your first and second sets as above, and do your third set of six to eight repetitions with twenty-pound dumbbells.

Remember, if the dumbbells are too heavy, go lighter, especially for the weaker muscles, such as the triceps and the shoulders. You may want to go as low as five, eight, and ten on these muscles for the first week or two. Don't rush it. You'll be amazed at how fast your muscles gain strength and how quickly you increase your weights. Let your body tell you what to do! Don't try to rush it, but on the other hand, don't hold it back. Listen carefully. Your body knows itself.

USING THE ALTERNATIVES

You will notice that almost every exercise offers an Alternative. Feel free to substitute them for the given exercise anytime you please. In some cases they involve a barbell, so you will not be able to do them unless you are willing to purchase one.

After you are working out for a few months, it's a good idea to take advantage of some of the alternatives, just to expand the variety of your workout. But you don't have to do it. You could just do the regular exercises forever, and you would get and stay in top shape!

STRETCHING

A lot of people wonder why there is no required stretching routine with any of my workouts. The answer is simple. There is a natural stretching system built into the workout. Your first set is light, and provides a natural stretch. If you go into any bodybuilding gym, you will notice that most bodybuilders never take time to do special stretches, although some do.

If you want to do special stretches, by all means do your own regular ones, or do one set of each exercise in the workout without weights before you start. In other words, go through the whole workout first, doing one quick set of each exercise with no weight. This will take you about five minutes. Again, some people view this as a waste of time, but you know your body. Do it if you feel that you should.

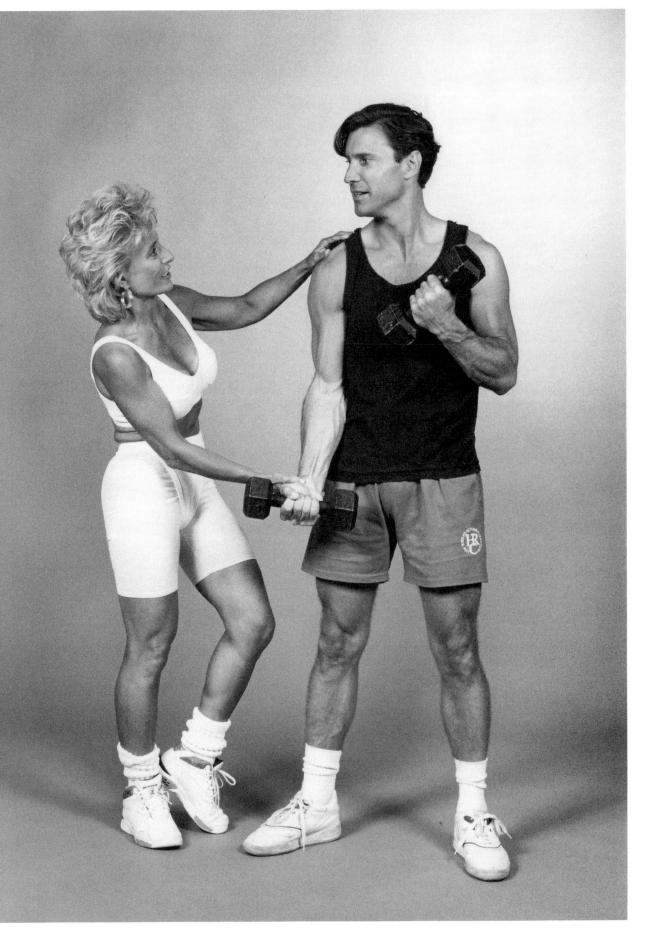

6

The Free Weight Workout

All of the exercises in this chapter are done with free weights—a few sets of dumbbells. Only some of the variations require barbells and plates—but there's no reason to feel obligated to try them unless you are so inclined. If you are working out in a gym, or using a home gym, go to Chapter 7. That workout offers the option of two to four machine exercises per body part (you will be asked to refer to this chapter for certain free weight exercises).

This chapter contains the **forty-minute, three-day plan**, and the **thirty-minute, four-day split routine**. If you choose the split routine, you can exercise up to six days a week if you so desire, because the system allows for an automatic day of rest between body parts. If, however, you choose the three-day plan, you cannot work out more than three days a week, or you will violate the forty-eight-hour rest principle. See pp. 4 and 43 for a review of this information.

FORTY-MINUTE, THREE-DAY PLAN
(DO ON EACH WORKOUT DAY)

chest
biceps
triceps
abdominals
back
shoulders

SPLIT ROUTINE WORKOUT DAYS ONE AND THREE	SPLIT ROUTINE WORKOUT DAYS TWO AND FOUR
chest	abdominals
biceps	back
triceps	shoulders
abdominals	thighs (optional)
	calves (optional)

(If you choose to exercise your legs, you will have to do the split routine—too much work for one day! See p. 43 for the discussion on this.)

This chapter will also include the optional Ironman and Superman routines, which ask you to add one or two exercises to each body part. If you are doing either of these routines, since you will be adding time to your workout, you may want to do a split routine, but if you have the energy, the choice is yours. You can still do the three-day workout! A review of this information is found on p. 58.

CHEST ROUTINE

1 • Flat Dumbbell Press

Increases strength and mass of the entire pectoral (chest) muscle, especially the outer area of the muscle.

Position: Lie on a flat exercise bench with your knees bent and your feet flat on the bench, or with your legs straddling the bench and your feet touching the floor on either side of the bench. Hold a dumbbell in each hand with your palms facing away from your body, and the outer edge of each dumbbell touching your outer chest area.

Movement: Flexing your pectoral muscles as you go, extend your arms upward, pressing the weights in balance with each other, until your arms are fully extended and the dumbbells are nearly touching each other at each end. Flex your pectoral muscles as hard as possible, and in full control, return to start position. Feel the stretch in your pectoral muscles and repeat the movement until you have completed your set.

Sets and Reps: See p. 54.

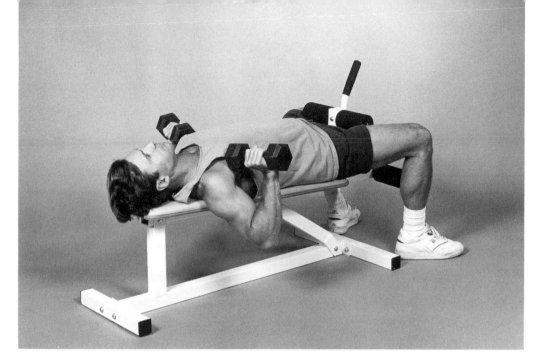

Start ———————————————————————————————————

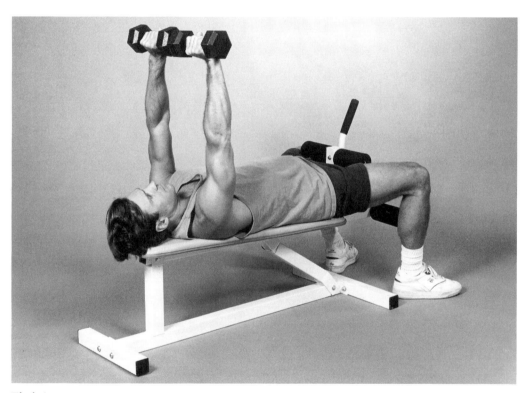

Finish ———————————————————————————————————

Tips: Don't hold your breath. Breathe naturally. Keep your mind riveted on your pectoral muscles throughout the exercise.

Alternatives: You may do this exercise with a barbell.

2 · Flat Dumbbell Flye

Develops, shapes, defines, and strengthens the entire pectoral (chest) muscle.

Position: Lie on a flat exercise bench with a dumbbell in each hand, palms facing each other. Extend your arms fully upward and let the dumbbells nearly touch each other.

Movement: Extend your arms outward and downward in a semicircle until you feel a full stretch in your chest (pectoral) muscles. Keep your wrists locked and slightly curled throughout the movement. In full control, return to start position, flexing your chest muscles as you go. Give your pectoral muscles an extra hard flex. Repeat the movement until you have completed your set.

Sets and
Reps: See p. 54.

Tips: Keep your elbows slightly bent throughout the movement. Don't hold your breath. Breathe naturally.

Alternatives: This exercise is sometimes replaced by the pec-deck machine exercise.

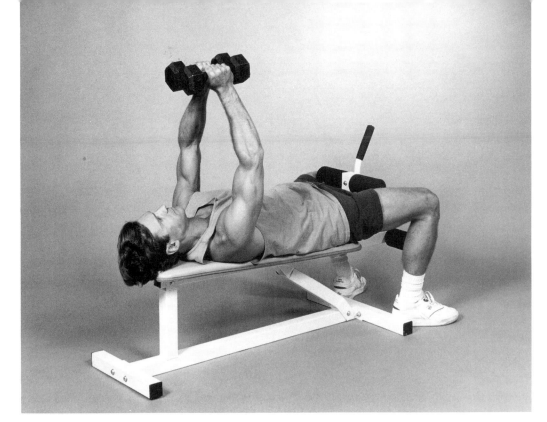

Start ——————————————————————————————

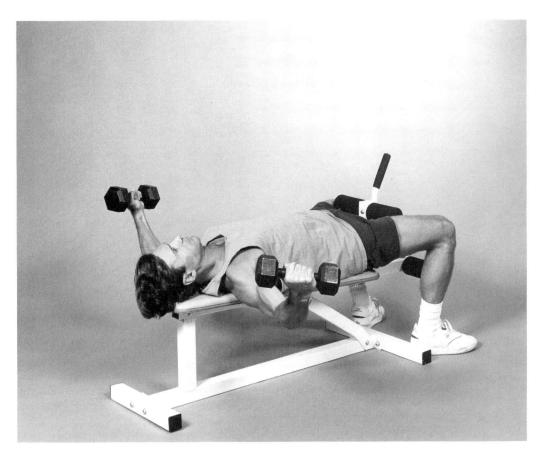

Finish ——————————————————————————————

77

3 • Incline Dumbbell Press

Develops, strengthens, and defines the upper pectoral (chest) area.

Position and Movement: Perform this exercise in exactly the same manner as the flat dumbbell press, but do it on an incline bench.

Sets and Reps: See p. 54.

Alternatives: This exercise can be done on a decline bench (a bench that tilts downward and has footholds). Done on a decline, the exercise develops the lower pectoral muscles.

4 • Incline Dumbbell Flye
(for Ironman and Superman workouts)

Develops, strengthens, and defines the upper pectoral (chest) muscle.

Position and Movement: Perform this exercise in exactly the same manner as the flat dumbbell flye, only do it on an incline bench.

Alternatives: This exercise can be replaced by the cable crossover, which is done on a cable crossover machine.

5 • Straight-Arm Cross-Bench Pullover
(for Superman workout)

Develops, shapes, defines, and strengthens the entire pectoral (chest) muscle and expands the rib cage. Also develops the serratus (upper side-chest) muscles.

Position: Place your shoulders at the edge of a flat exercise bench with your head extended over the bench, and your feet flat on the floor. Keep your buttocks low to the ground. Hold the dumbbell with both hands, palms against the underside of the top plate, so that the stem of the plate fits between your thumb and fingers. Hold the dumbbell with arms extended straight up, directly above your midchest area.

Movement: Bending your elbows the least amount possible, extend your arms behind you, lowering the weight in an arc behind you, keeping your buttocks low to the floor and letting your arms descend as low as possible, until you feel a full stretch in your chest and rib cage. Flexing your pectoral muscles as you go, return to start position. Give your pectoral muscles an extra hard flex. Repeat the movement until you have completed your set.

Tips: Keep your elbows as straight as possible throughout the movement.

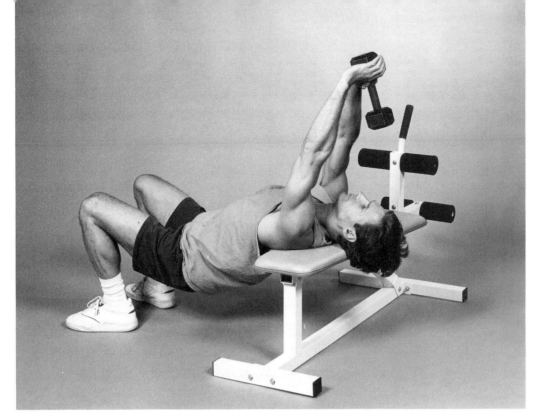

Start —————————————————

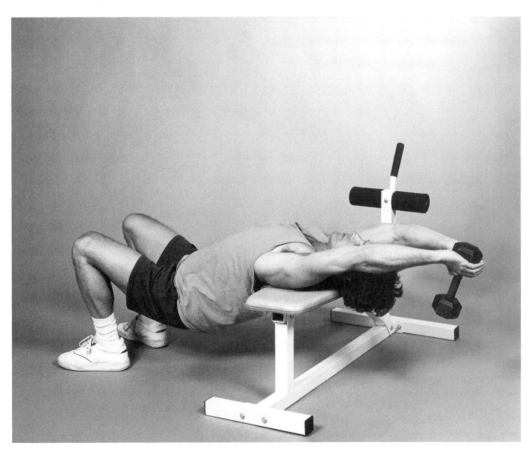

Finish —————————————————

81

BICEPS ROUTINE

1 • Seated Simultaneous Dumbbell Curl with a Twist

Strengthens and develops the entire biceps, and gives the biceps shape and definition.

Position: Sit at the edge of a flat exercise bench with a dumbbell in each hand, your arms straight down at your sides, palms facing your body.

Movement: In one movement, twisting your wrists so that your palms are facing in front of you, and flexing your biceps muscles as you go, curl both dumbbells upward simultaneously, keeping your elbows close to your body, until the dumbbells are at your shoulders, or as far as your curling arms will allow them to go. Flex your biceps as hard as possible, and return to start. Feel the stretch in your biceps muscles and repeat the movement until you have completed your set.

Sets and Reps: See p. 55.

Tips: Keep your elbows close to your sides throughout the movement.

Alternatives: For greater stretch and elongation, perform this exercise while lying on an incline bench. You may perform this exercise alternating arms, or standing, with a barbell.

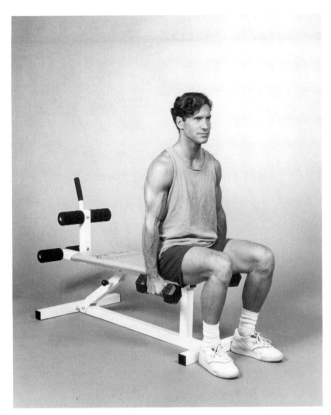

Start —————————————————

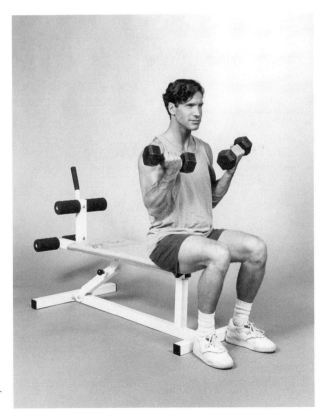

Finish —————————————

2 · Seated Alternate Hammer Curl

Develops, shapes, strengthens, and defines the biceps muscle and the forearm.

Position: Sit at the edge of a flat exercise bench with a dumbbell held in each hand, palms facing your body and arms straight down at your sides.

Movement: With dumbbells in the "hammer" position (see photograph), flexing your left biceps as you go, curl your left arm up toward your left shoulder. As the dumbbell approaches your left shoulder, flexing your right biceps as you go, begin curling your right arm up toward your right shoulder; at the same time, uncurl your left arm. Continue this alternate curl movement until you have completed your set.

Sets and Reps: See p. 55.

Tips: Give your biceps muscle an extra hard flex each time your arm reaches the highest peak of the curl, and let your biceps muscle fully stretch out on the down position. Do not rock back and forth. Let your biceps do the work, not your shoulders or your back.

Alternatives: You may perform this exercise standing.

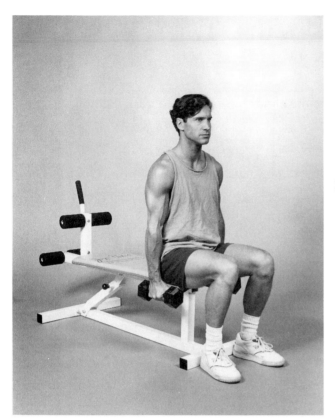

Start ─────────────────────

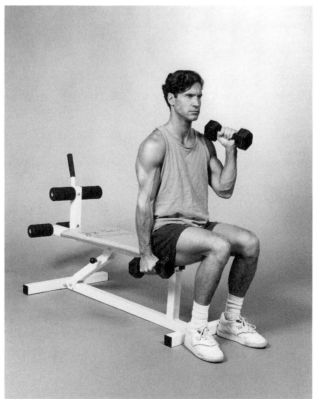

Finish ─────────────────────

3 • Concentration Curl with a Twist

Develops, shapes, strengthens, and defines the entire biceps muscle, especially the peak and the outside area.

Position:	With your heels about two feet apart, bend over and position your right elbow on your right inner knee, holding a dumbbell with your palm facing away from your body and your arm extended straight down. Place your other arm on your knee or at your side in order to steady yourself.
Movement:	Keeping your upper arm steady, and flexing your biceps muscle as you go, curl the dumbbell up until it reaches shoulder height, and twist your wrist so that your pinky finger is higher than your thumb. Flex your biceps muscle as hard as possible, and return to start position. Feel the stretch in your biceps muscle. Repeat the movement until you have completed your set. Repeat the set for your other arm.
Sets and Reps:	See p. 55.
Tips:	Do not let your elbow wander away from your knee area as you work. Don't hold your breath. Breathe naturally.
Alternatives:	This exercise can be done seated.

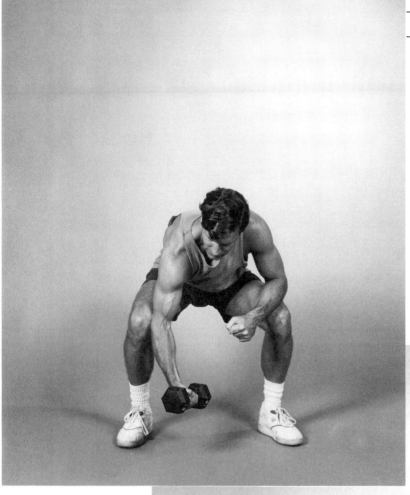

Start

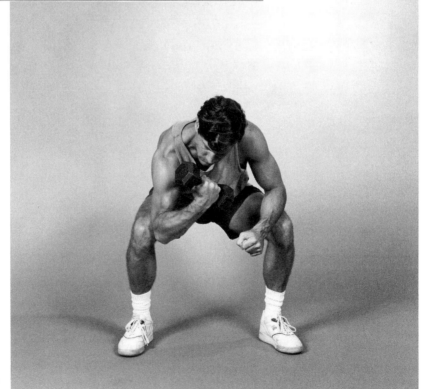

Finish

4 • Lying Alternate Dumbbell Curl
(for Ironman and Superman workouts)

Develops, shapes, strengthens, and defines the entire biceps muscle, especially the peak.

Position: With a dumbbell in each hand, palms facing upward, lie on your back on a flat exercise bench. Let your arms extend fully downward so that you can feel the full stretch in your biceps muscle. Your feet should be nearly flat on the floor.

Movement: Keeping your palm facing upward, and flexing your biceps muscle as you go, curl your right arm up toward your shoulder, and just when that dumbbell reaches shoulder height, flex your biceps muscle as hard as possible and begin to curl your left arm upward; at the same time, begin to uncurl your right biceps. Return your right arm to start position and feel the full stretch in that muscle. Continue to do this alternate curling movement until you have completed your set.

Tips: Keep your elbows close to your body. Don't let your body rise from the bench. Curl the dumbbells up as high as possible. Don't hold your breath. Breathe naturally.

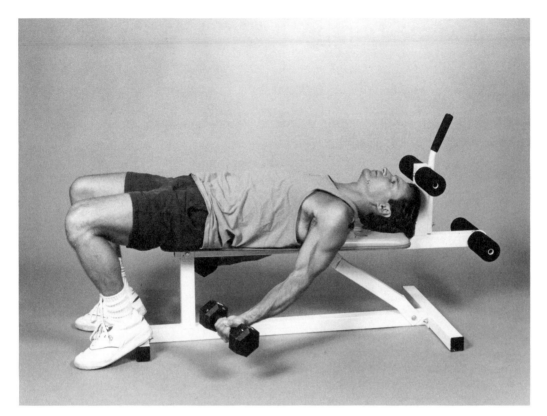

Start

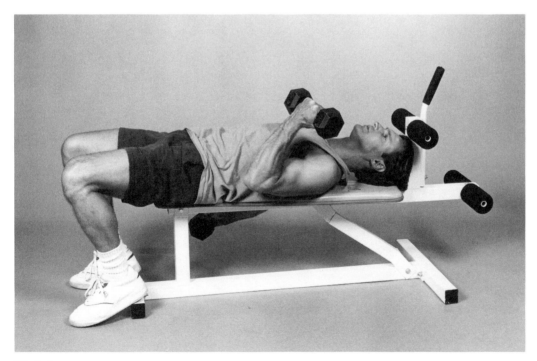

Finish

5 • Reverse Dumbbell Curl
(for Superman workout)

Develops, strengthens, shapes, and defines the entire biceps muscle, especially the outer area, and helps to build the forearm.

Position: Stand with your feet a natural width apart, with a dumbbell in each hand, palms facing your body, and with your thumbs on the upper edge of the bar of the dumbbell. Your arms should be straight down at your sides—but slightly in front of you.

Movement: Keeping your upper arms as close to your body as possible, and flexing your biceps and forearms as you go, curl your arms upward until your fists reach approximately chin height. Flex your biceps and forearms as hard as possible, and return to start position. Feel the stretch in your biceps, and repeat the movement until you have completed your set.

Tips: Do not let your elbows wander away from your body. Keep your thumbs on top of the bar of the dumbbell in order to challenge the outer area of your biceps muscle.

Alternatives: You may perform this exercise by alternating arms. You may use a barbell instead of dumbbells.

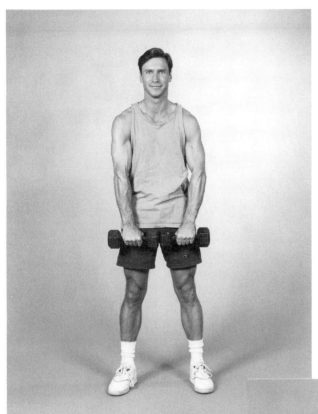

Start

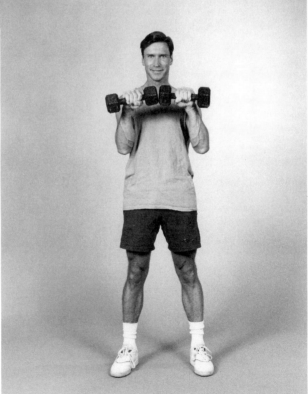

Finish

TRICEPS ROUTINE

1 • Lying Dumbbell Extension

Develops, strengthens, shapes, and defines the entire triceps muscle, especially the outer triceps area.

Position: Lie on a flat exercise bench with your knees bent, and the soles of your feet flat on the floor, holding a dumbbell in each hand, palms facing each other. Extend your arms straight up so that the dumbbells are centered above each pectoral muscle.

Movement: Keeping your elbows steady and as stationary as possible, bending at the elbows, simultaneously lower the dumbbells until the dumbbells reach your shoulders. Feel the stretch in your triceps muscles and, flexing your triceps muscles as you go, return to start position, locking your elbows. Flex your triceps muscles as hard as possible and repeat the movement until you have completed your set.

Sets and
Reps: See p. 55.

Tips: Keep your elbows in line with your body throughout the movement. Do not let them wander out. Don't hold your breath. Breathe naturally.

Alternatives: You may perform this exercise one arm at a time by alternating the dumbbells.

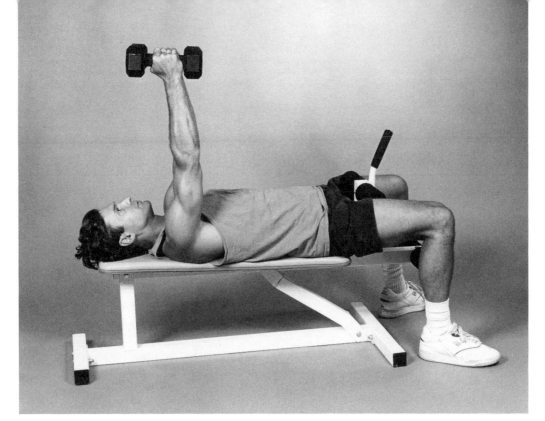

Start ————————————————————————————————

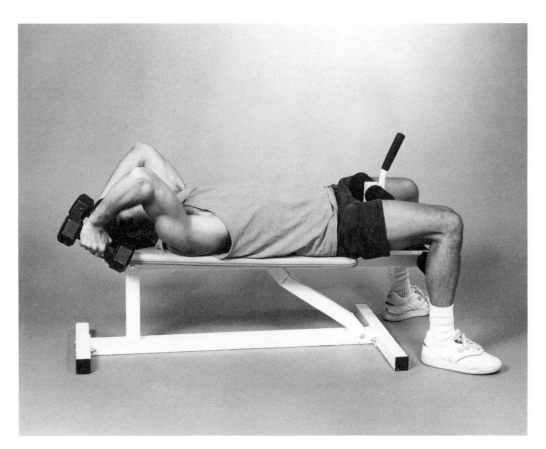

Finish ————————————————————————————————

2 • One-Arm Triceps Kickback with a Twist

Develops, shapes, strengthens, and defines the entire triceps muscle, especially the upper area.

Position:
: With a dumbbell held in your left hand, palm facing your body, bend at the waist and stand with your knees bent, and with one foot slightly in front of the other. Keep your elbow about an inch above your waist area, and close to your body throughout the exercise.

Movement:
: Keeping your left arm close to your body, and flexing your triceps muscle as you go, extend your left arm back as far as possible. As you reach the furthest point, twist your wrist slightly by raising your thumb so that your palm is almost facing behind you, and at the same time, flex your triceps muscle as hard as possible. Return to start position and feel the stretch in your triceps muscle. Repeat the movement until you have completed your set. Repeat the set for your other arm.

Sets and Reps:
: See p. 55.

Tips:
: Your upper arm must remain close to your body at all times during the movement.

Alternatives:
: This movement can be performed two arms at a time.

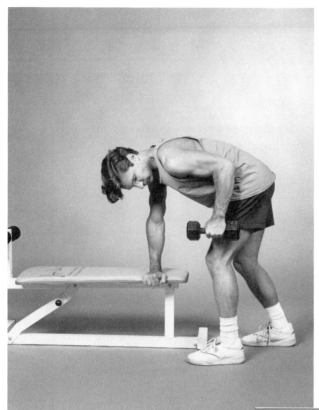

Start

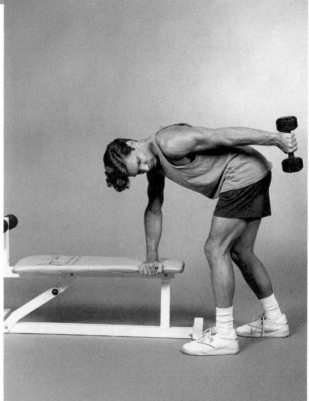

Finish

3 • Seated One-Arm Triceps Overhead Extension with a Twist

Develops, shapes, strengthens, and defines all three heads of the triceps muscle, especially the inner and medial heads of that muscle.

Position: Sit on a flat exercise bench holding a dumbbell in your right hand, palm facing front and your arm extended straight up so that your biceps is nearly touching your ear.

Movement: Twist your wrist toward your body and lower the dumbbell behind your head until you cannot go any further (the end of the dumbbell should touch the back of your neck), and feel the stretch in your triceps muscle. Untwist your wrist so that your palm is facing away from you as you raise the dumbbell to start position. Flex your triceps muscle as hard as possible and return to start position. Repeat the movement until you have completed your set. Repeat the movement for your other arm.

Sets and
Reps: See p. 55.

Tips: Keep your upper arm close to your body throughout the movement. Do not hold your breath. Breathe naturally.

Alternatives: You can perform this exercise two arms at a time, using one dumbbell (heavier, of course).

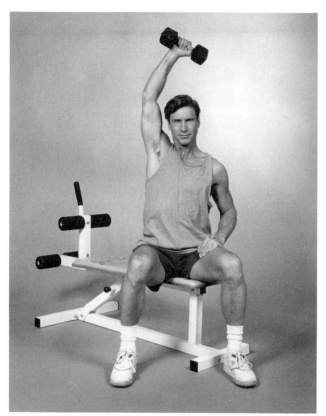

Start ——————————

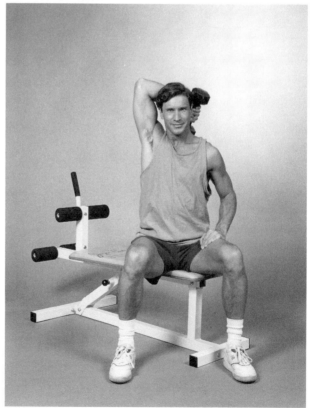

Finish ——————————

4 • Cross-Face Triceps Extension
(for Ironman and Superman workouts)

Develops, shapes, strengthens, and defines the entire triceps muscle.

Position: Lie on a flat exercise bench with a dumbbell held in your right hand, palm facing your body. Extend your right arm upward until your elbow is locked. Turn your face away from the dumbbell.

Movement: Feeling the stretch in your right triceps muscle as you go, bend your right arm at the elbow, and lower your arm until the dumbbell touches your left neck-shoulder area. Flexing your right triceps muscle as you go, return to start position. Give your right triceps muscle an extra hard flex and return to start position. Repeat the movement until you have completed your set. Repeat the set for your other arm.

Tips: Do not let your arm wander away from your head as you work. Don't let the dumbbell nearly drop down to your ear, or jerk it up to start position. Maintain control at all times. Don't hold your breath. Breathe naturally.

Alternatives: This exercise can be done on an incline bench.

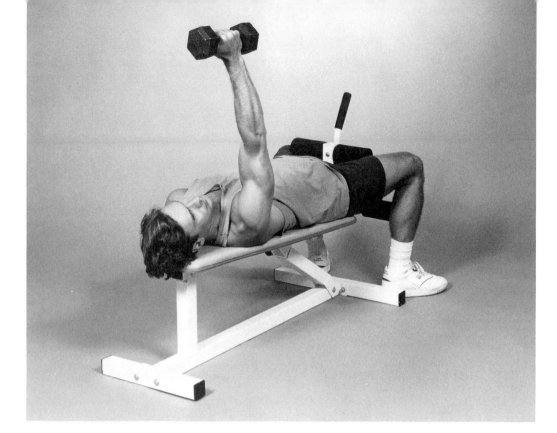

Start

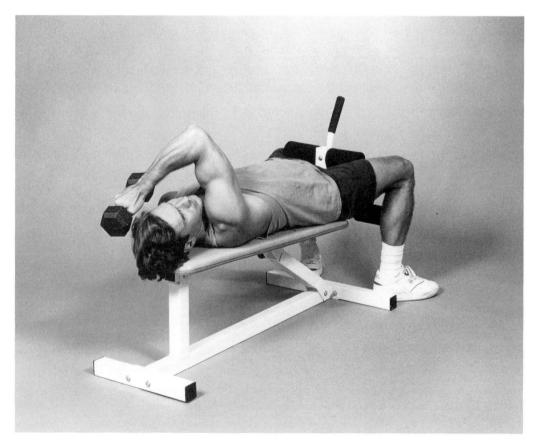

Finish

5 • Dips Between Benches
(for Superman workout)

Develops, shapes, strengthens, and defines the entire triceps muscle, especially the elbow area, and adds thickness to the entire muscle.

Position: Line up two flat exercise benches so that they are parallel to each other and wide enough apart so that when you lean on one with the palms of your hands, the heels of your feet just fit on the edge of the other without falling off. (You may use blocks of wood or any device where you can rest your heels.) Your heels should be about the same height as your arms or higher. With your palms flat on the bench and about shoulder-width apart, curl your fingers around the bench for support and hold yourself up with your fully extended arms.

Movement: Bending at the elbows, lower your body as far down as possible. Without resting, and using the strength of your triceps muscles, raise your body to start position and flex your triceps muscles as hard as possible. Repeat the movement until you have completed your set.

Tips: Once you have gotten used to the exercise, you may place a dumbbell on your lap—raising the weight of the dumbbell for each set, just as you do for all other exercises. Beware of the temptation to cut the movement short by not lowering yourself all the way.

Alternatives: This exercise can be performed on any dips bar device found in most fitness centers.

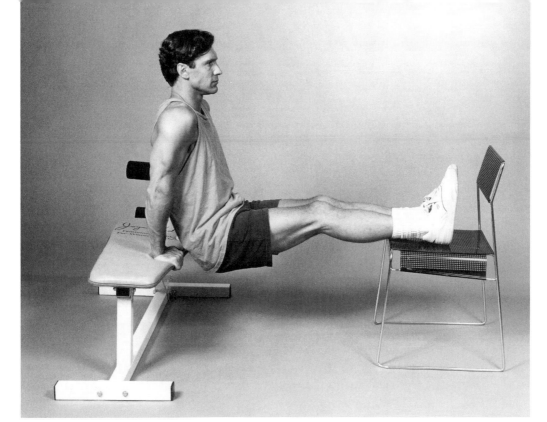

Start

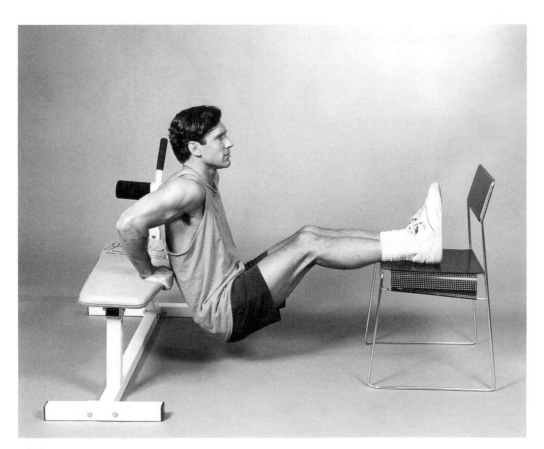

Finish

101

ABDOMINAL ROUTINE

1 • Alternate Knee-in

Develops, shapes, strengthens, and defines the lower abdominal muscles and slightly challenges the upper abdominal area.

Position:	Lie on the floor with your legs extended straight out in front of you, but about three inches off the floor. Place the palms of your hands flat on the floor and under each buttock. Support yourself on your elbows.
Movement:	Flexing your abdominal muscles as you go, bending at the knee, bring your left knee as close to your left shoulder as possible. Flex your left lower abdominal muscles as hard as possible and then begin to straighten your left leg, while at the same time beginning to bend your right knee, bringing it to your right shoulder. Continue this bicycle-like movement, remembering to give your abdominal muscles an extra hard flex each time a knee reaches approximate shoulder height.
Sets and Reps:	See p. 56.
Tips:	One leg should be up while the other is down throughout this exercise. Imagine that you are riding a bicycle, only remember to flex each time on the up movement.
Alternatives:	You can perform this movement by placing your hands behind your head and twisting from side to side—having your right knee meet your left shoulder, and so on. This method will challenge your oblique muscles in addition to your lower abdominals.

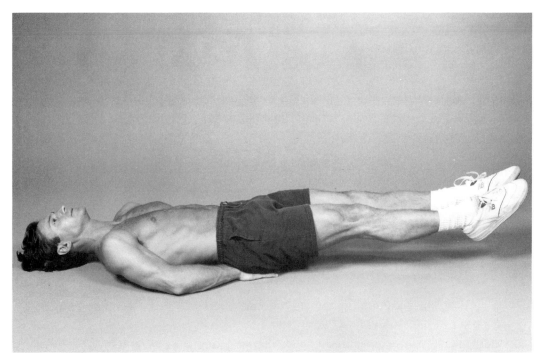

Start

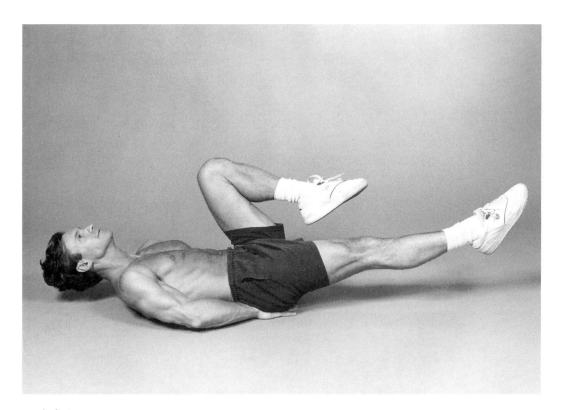

Finish

2 • Knee-Raised Crunch

Develops, shapes, strengthens, and defines the upper abdominal muscles and helps to strengthen the lower abdominal muscles.

Position:
Lie flat on your back with your knees fully bent and your ankles crossed and in the air.

Movement:
Flexing your abdominal muscles as you go, raise your head and shoulders off the ground, moving toward your knees as far as possible, without lifting your back off the ground. Give your abdominals an extra hard flex, and return to start position. Feel the stretch in your abdominal muscles and repeat the movement until you have completed your set.

Sets and Reps:
See p. 56.

Tips:
This is not a sit-up. Do not raise your upper body to more than a shoulders-off-the-ground position.

Alternatives:
You may perform this exercise by twisting your body from side to side as you crunch. In this case, you would alternately aim your right elbow toward your left knee, and your left elbow toward your right knee as you crunch.

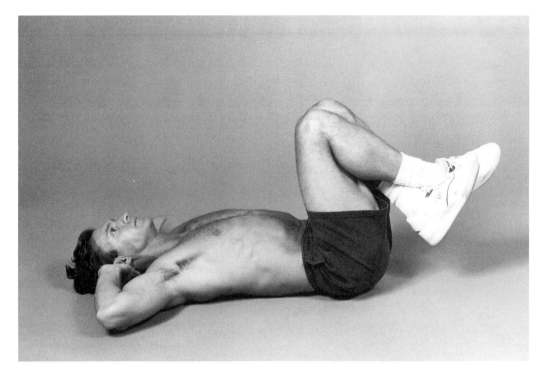

Start

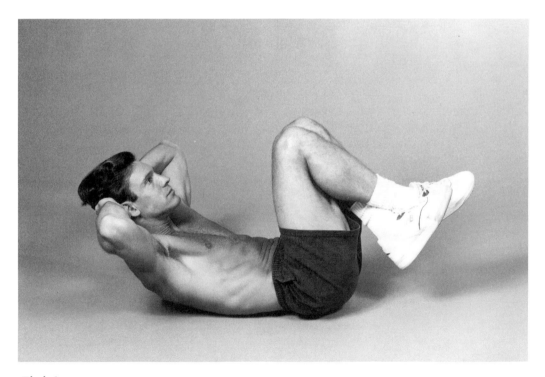

Finish

3 • Squatting Side Bend

Develops, shapes, strengthens, and defines the oblique (side abdominal) muscles.

Position: Stand with your feet a foot wider than shoulder-width apart, bending at the knee until you are nearly in a squatting position. Place your hands behind your head and keep them there by interlacing your fingers.

Movement: Bending at the waist, and flexing your left oblique (side abdominal) muscles as you go, bring your left elbow to your right knee. Give your left oblique muscles an extra hard flex, and without resting, return to start position and repeat the movement for the other side of your body.

Sets and
Reps: See p. 56.

Tips: Keep your mind riveted on your oblique muscles as you work. Remember to flex them as hard as possible in each downward position.

Alternatives: Beware of those who will tell you that you can do this by standing, holding a weight in each hand, and bending from side to side. Doing this movement with weight will add mass to the oblique muscles, and will make your waist thicker—the last thing you want to have happen!

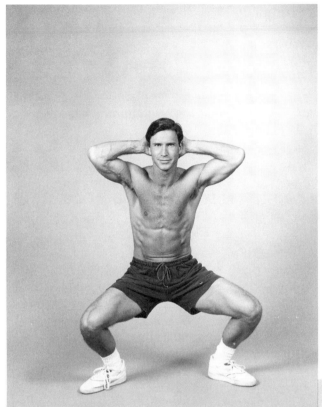

Start —————————————

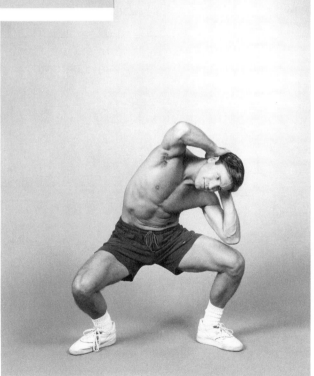

Finish —————————————————

4 • Reverse Crunch
(for Ironman and Superman workouts)

Develops, shapes, strengthens, and defines the lower abdominal muscles and strengthens the lower back.

Position: Lie on the floor flat on your back with your knees completely bent (to an approximate 90 degree angle). Place your hands behind your head and point your knees toward the ceiling.

Movement: Keeping your knees together and pointed toward the ceiling, and flexing your lower abdominal muscles as you go, raise your lower abdominal area by lifting your pelvis and bringing your knees as close to your chest as possible. In this high position, flex your lower abdominal muscles as hard as possible and return to start position. Feel the stretch in your lower abdominal muscles. Repeat the movement until you have completed your set.

Tips: At first it may seem as if you are jerking your body to the up position, but in time you will gain more control and find that you are able to perform the exercise in a more fluid manner. Don't hold your breath. Breathe naturally.

Alternatives: You may substitute this exercise for the standard leg raise.

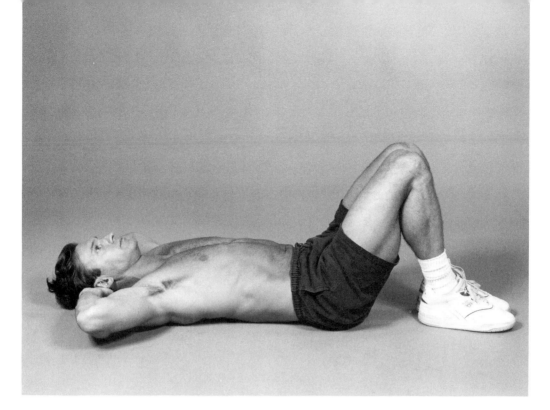

Start

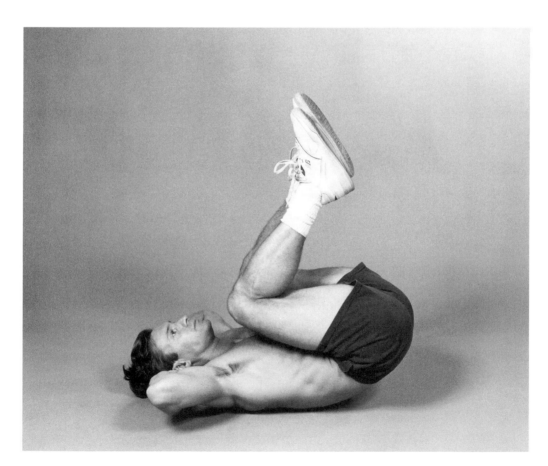

Finish

5 • Knee-Raised Twisting Sit-up

(for Superman workout)

Develops, shapes, strengthens, and defines upper, lower, and oblique (side) abdominal muscles.

Position: Lie flat on your back on the floor with your hands behind your head. Raise your knees to an approximate 90 degree angle, and cross your legs at the ankles. Mentally anchor your buttocks to the floor.

Movement: Flexing your entire abdominal area as you go, sit up and at the same time twist your body by bringing your left elbow to your left knee. In the highest position, flex your left abdominal muscles as hard as possible and return to start position, and without hesitation, repeat the movement for the other side of your body. Continue this alternative movement until you have completed the designated number of repetitions for each side of your body.

Tips: If the movement is too difficult, you may perform it without the twist and with your arms extended out in front of you. (Naturally, your abdominals will not get the same amount of challenge, but later you can advance to the more difficult movement.)

Alternatives: You can replace this exercise with the standard bent-knee sit-up.

Notes: If you are following a split routine, stop here. Your workout days one and three are over. If you are following a three-day-a-week workout plan, continue on and do your back and shoulders.

For additional alternatives to all abdominal exercises, see bibliography for *Gut Busters*.

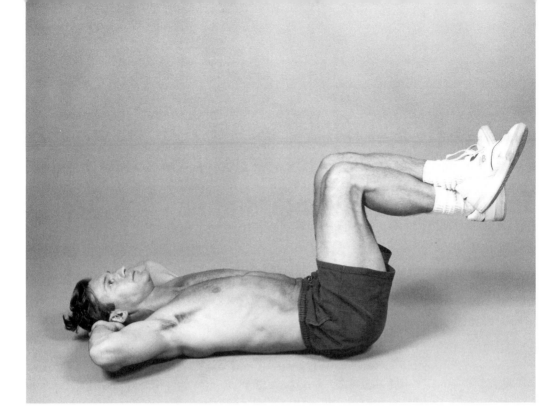

Start —————————————————————————————————

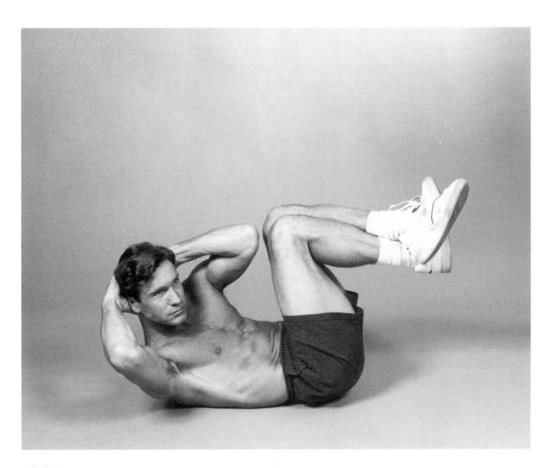

Finish —————————————————————————————————

111

BACK ROUTINE

1 • Double-Arm Bent Dumbbell Row

Develops, shapes, strengthens and defines the latissimus dorsi and upper back muscles.

Position: With a dumbbell in each hand, palms facing your body, and your feet a natural width apart, bend over until your torso is nearly parallel to the floor. Your knees should be slightly bent, and your arms should be hanging straight down, in line with your shoulders, the dumbbells held close to your body. Keep your head up.

Movement: Keeping your upper body stable, and flexing your lat and upper back muscles as you go, raise the dumbbells in unison until they reach your waist area. Flex your upper back muscles as hard as possible. Return to start position and feel a full stretch in your lat and upper back muscles. Repeat the movement until you have completed your set.

Sets and
Reps: See p. 56.

Tips: Maintain full control of the dumbbells throughout the exercise. Don't jerk them up or let them drop down.

Alternatives: You may perform this exercise with a barbell held in front of you.

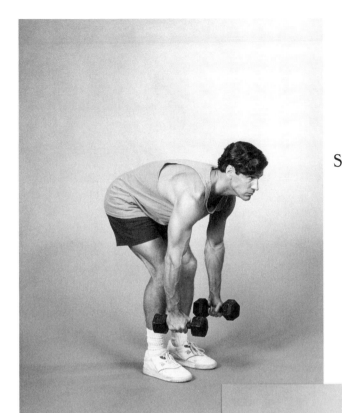

Start

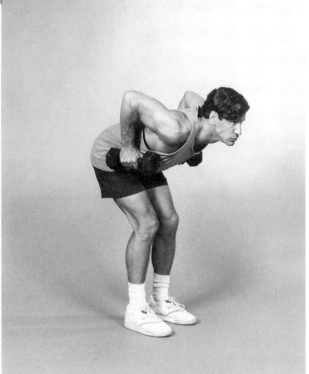

Finish

2 • Single-Arm Bent Dumbbell Row

Develops, shapes, strengthens, and defines the latissumus dorsi and center back muscles.

Position: Stand near a flat exercise bench, and lean on the bench with your right hand, holding a dumbbell, palm facing your body with your left hand. Bend at the waist until your upper body is nearly parallel to the floor. Let your left arm hang down, fully extended, and let the weight completely stretch your left upper back muscles.

Movement: Raise your left arm, keeping it close to your body, flexing your upper back muscles as you go, and using your upper back rather than your arm muscles to do the work. Raise your elbow as high as possible and flex your left upper back muscles as hard as possible. Without rocking from side to side, return to start position and feel the full stretch in your left upper back muscles. Repeat the movement until you have completed your set. Repeat the exercise for the other side of your back.

Sets and
Reps: See p. 56.

Tips: Do not jerk the weight up or nearly let it drop down. Maintain full control at all times.

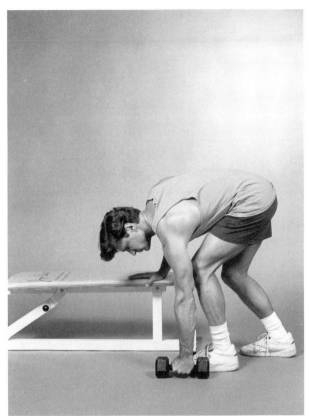

Start

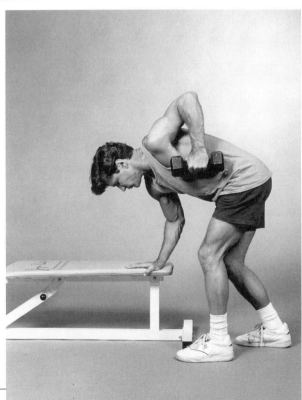

Finish

3 • Upright Row

Develops, shapes, strengthens, and defines the trapezius muscles. Also helps to shape the front deltoid (shoulder) muscle.

Position: Stand with your feet a natural width apart and hold a dumbbell with both hands in the center, your palms facing your body. Extend your arms fully downward. The dumbbell should be centered in front of your upper thigh area.

Movement: Flexing your trapezius muscles as you go, extending your elbows outward, and keeping the dumbbell close to your body, raise the dumbbell until it reaches chin height. Flex your trapezius muscles as hard as possible and return to start position. Feel the stretch in your trapezius muscles. Repeat the movement until you have completed your set.

Sets and   See p. 56.
Reps:

Tips: Keep the weight close to your body as you raise and lower your arms. It is a little awkward doing the exercise with a dumbbell because of the width of the dumbbell plates, so you will have to be careful to force the dumbbell to stay close to your body.

Alternatives: You may perform this exercise with a barbell.

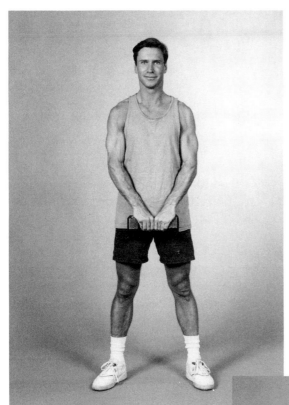

Start ————————————————

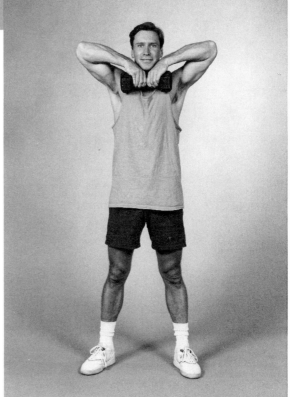

Finish ————————————————

4 • Dumbbell Deadlift Shrug
(for Ironman and Superman workouts)

Develops, shapes, strengthens, and defines the lower back and the trapezius muscles.

Position: Stand with your feet a natural width apart and hold a dumbbell in each hand, palms facing your body. Bend at the knees, holding the weights in front of your toes, but a few inches to either side. Let the weights touch the ground but do not let go of them.

Movement: Rise from the squatting position with the strength of your legs, and as you are nearly standing upright, pull your shoulders up and curl them back and down in a shrugging movement. Let the dumbbells hang in your hands as weights. Return to start position and repeat the movement until you have completed your set.

Tips: Be sure to bend at the knees. Do not merely lean forward, or you will hurt your back.

Alternatives: You may perform this exercise with a barbell.

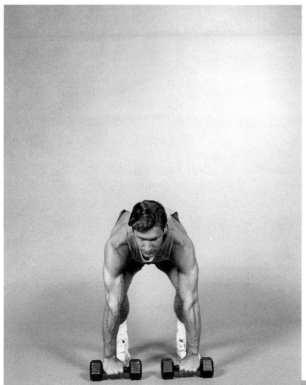

Start

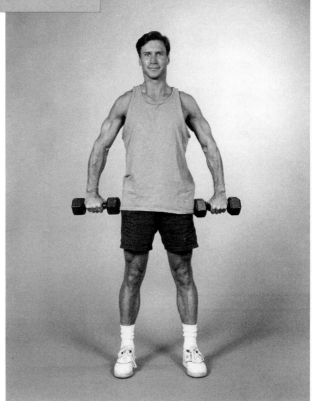

Finish

5 • Seated Dumbbell Back Lateral
(for Superman workout)

Develops, shapes, strengthens, and defines the upper back and trapezius muscles.

Position: While holding a dumbbell in each hand, sit at the edge of a flat exercise bench and lean forward until your upper body is nearly parallel to the floor. Hold the dumbbells with your palms facing away from you behind your ankles. Let the dumbbells touch each other at the ends.

Movement: Flexing your upper back muscles as you go, and keeping the dumbbells close to your legs at all times, raise the dumbbells up and back, rotating the dumbbells as you go along. When you reach hip level, your palms are facing away from your body and either side of each dumbbell is about three to four inches from your hip area. Flex your upper back muscles as hard as possible by pretending to try to squeeze a pencil in the center of your back. Return to start position, feeling the stretch in your upper back muscles. Repeat the movement until you have completed your set.

Tips: Keep the dumbbells as close to your body as possible throughout the movement. Don't hold your breath. Breathe naturally.

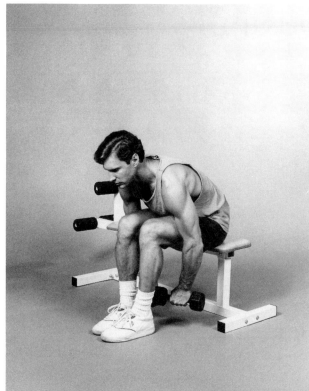

Start

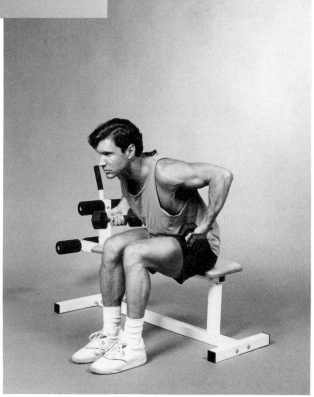

Finish

SHOULDER ROUTINE

1 • Seated Simultaneous Dumbbell Press

Develops, strengthens, shapes, and defines the entire deltoid (shoulder) muscle, especially the front area.

Position: Sit on a flat exercise bench with a dumbbell held in each hand at shoulder height, palms facing away from your body.

Movement: Flexing your shoulder muscles as you go, raise the dumbbells simultaneously and let them nearly touch at the top (at this point your arms will be almost fully extended upward). Flex your shoulder muscles as hard as possible and return to start position. Feel the stretch in your shoulder muscles, and repeat the movement until you have completed your set.

Sets and   See p. 57.
Reps:

Tips: Maintain control of the dumbbells at all times. Don't merely jerk them up or let them nearly drop down to start position. Keep your mind riveted on your front shoulder muscles as you work.

Alternatives: You may perform this exercise one arm at a time. You may perform this exercise with a barbell behind your neck.

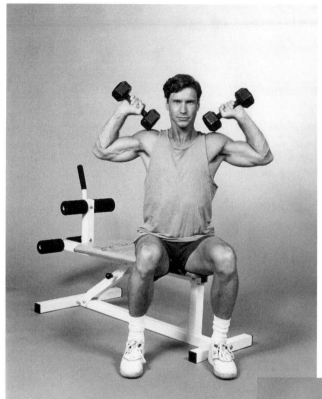

Start

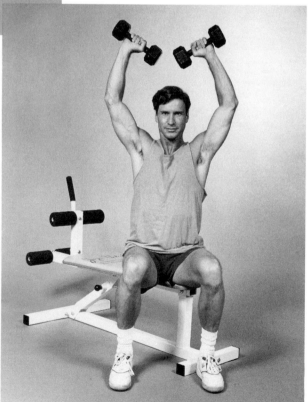

Finish

2 • Seated Side Lateral

Develops, shapes, strengthens, and defines the entire deltoid (shoulder) muscle, especially the side area.

Position: Sit on a flat exercise bench with a dumbbell in each hand, with your palms facing each other, and the dumbbells held in front of you in the center of your body.

Movement: Flexing your shoulder muscles as you go, simultaneously extend your arms outward and upward until the dumbbells are slightly higher than shoulder height. Flex your shoulder muscles as hard as possible and return to start position. Feel the stretch in your shoulder muscles and repeat the movement until you have completed your set.

Sets and Reps: See p. 57.

Tips: Beware of the temptation to swing the dumbbells out and to nearly let them drop to start position. Maintain control at all times. Keep your mind on your shoulder muscles. Don't hold your breath. Breathe naturally.

Alternatives: You may perform this exercise one arm at at time.

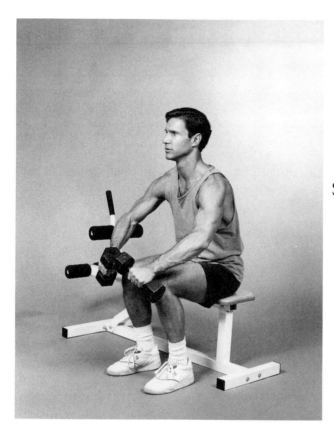

Start

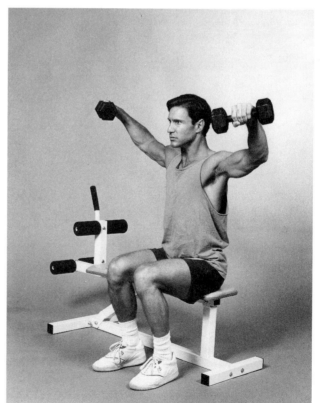

Finish

3 • Standing Bent Lateral with a Twist

Develops, shapes, strengthens, and defines the entire deltoid (shoulder) muscle, especially the rear and side areas.

Position: Stand with your feet together, holding a dumbbell in each hand, with palms facing each other. Bend over until your upper body is parallel to the floor and extend your arms straight down in front of you in the center of your body. Allow the dumbbells to touch each other.

Movement: Flexing your shoulder muscles as you go, keeping your body steady, and turning your wrists (your thumb will begin to descend), extend your arms out to the side, lifting the weights until your arms are parallel to the floor. (Your elbows will be very slightly bent and your thumb will be positioned lower than your pinky.) Flex your shoulder muscles as hard as possible, and keeping your arms in line with your shoulders, return to start position. Feel the stretch in your shoulder area, and repeat the movement until you have completed your set.

Sets and
Reps: See p. 57.

Tips: Do not let your upper body rise from the parallel-to-the-floor position throughout the exercise.

Alternatives: You may perform this exercise seated by positioning the dumbbells behind your calves.

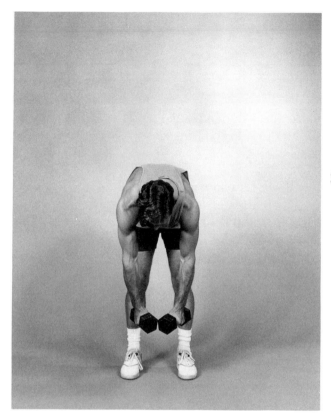

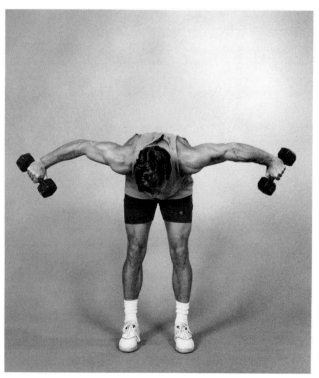

Finish

4 • Reverse Overhead Dumbbell Lateral
(for Ironman and Superman workouts)

Develops, shapes, strengthens, and defines the entire deltoid (shoulder) muscle, especially the front area, and helps to develop the trapezius muscles.

Position: Stand with your feet a natural width apart with a dumbbell in each hand, palms upward. Extend your arms out to either side so that they are nearly parallel to the floor. Curl your wrists upward and bend your elbows slightly.

Movement: Raise your arms up until the dumbbells meet over your head. Your elbows should remain slightly bent at the top position. Feel the stretch in your shoulder muscles. Return to start position and flex your shoulder muscles as hard as possible. Repeat the movement until you have completed your set.

Tips: In order to get the full benefit of this exercise, move slowly as you lower your arms to start position, resisting the weight as you go.

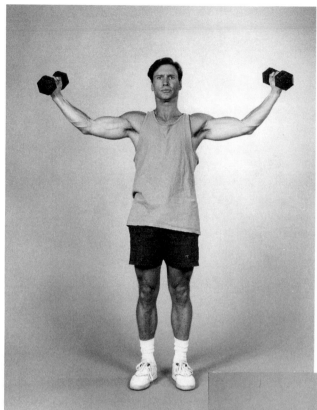

Start

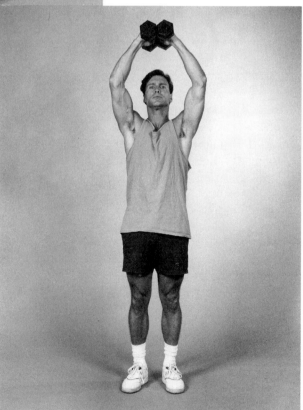

Finish

5 • Pee-Wee Lateral
(for Superman workout)

Develops, shapes, strengthens, and defines the rear and side deltoid (shoulder) muscles.

Position: Stand with your feet together, holding a dumbbell in each hand with palms facing away from your body and your arms behind your back. The ends of the dumbbells should be touching each other. Bend your knees slightly and thrust your hips forward.

Movement: Extend your arms outward and upward until the dumbbells reach ear height and are at arm's length on either side. Flex your shoulder muscles as hard as possible. Return to start position and feel the stretch in your shoulder muscles. Repeat the movement until you have completed your set.

Tips: Keep your body steady throughout the exercise. Do not rock back and forth. Don't hold your breath. Breathe naturally.

Stop! If you are doing a three-day routine, your workout is completed. Congratulations.

Go! If you are doing a split routine, you must now do your abdominals for workout day two and if in addition you are doing the optional leg workout, after you do back and shoulders, you must now proceed to do your thigh and calf routines.

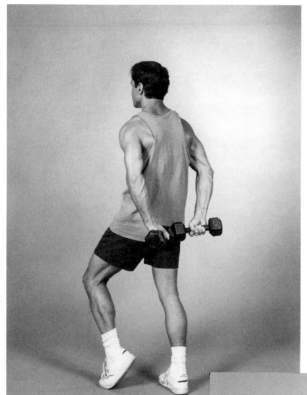

Start ————————————

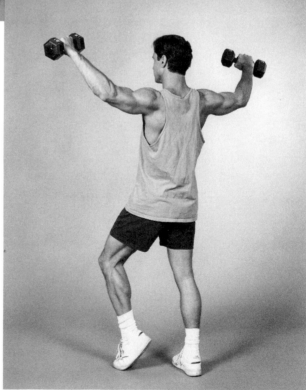

Finish ————————————

THIGH ROUTINE

(Workout days two and four for those who choose the optional leg workout)

1 • Regular Dumbbell Squat

Develops, shapes, strengthens, and defines the quadriceps (front thigh) muscles and helps to shape and tighten the gluteus maximus (buttocks) and hamstrings (back thigh) muscles.

Position: With a dumbbell held in each hand, palms facing your body, stand with your feet a natural width apart and your toes pointed slightly outward. Let your arms hang down at your sides. Keep your back straight and your eyes straight ahead.

Movement: Descend until your thighs are parallel to the floor, if your knees allow it; otherwise go as far as you can go, and feel a full stretch in your front thigh muscles as you reach the final position. Without resting or bouncing, and flexing your quadriceps (front thigh) muscles as you go, return to start position and flex your thigh and buttocks muscles as hard as possible. Repeat the movement until you have completed your set.

Tips: You may place a piece of wood under your heels for balance. Don't hold your breath. Breathe naturally.

Alternatives: You may perform this movement with a barbell placed behind your neck. You will need to use a squat rack, a barbell, and plates if you are planning to put significant size on your thighs, which will require heavy squatting (see p. 65 for more information on putting on size).

132

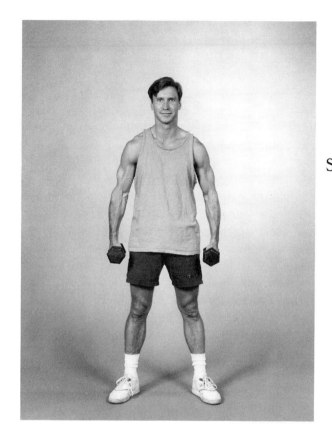

Start ———————————————

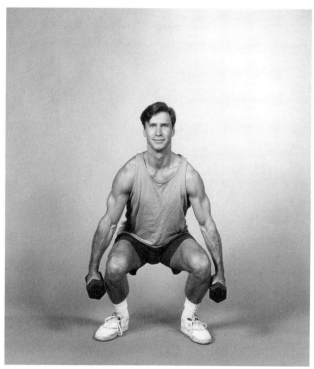

Finish ——————————————

2 • Narrow Dumbbell Squat

Develops, shapes, defines, and strengthens the quadriceps (outer thigh) area and helps to shape and tighten the gluteus maximus (buttocks) and hamstrings (back thigh) muscles.

Position: With a dumbbell held in each hand, palms facing your body, stand with your feet about four inches apart, toes pointed almost straight ahead. Let your arms hang down at your sides. Keep your back straight and your eyes straight ahead.

Movement: Descend until your thighs are parallel to the floor if your knees will allow it; otherwise go until you feel a full stretch in your thigh muscle—but do not endanger your knees. Without bouncing, and flexing your quadriceps (outer thigh) muscles as hard as possible, return to start position and repeat the movement until you have completed your set.

Tips: You may place a piece of wood under your heels for balance. Avoid the tendency to lean forward as you descend to the lower position. Keep your back erect throughout the movement.

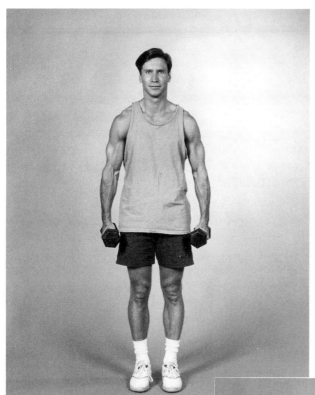

Start

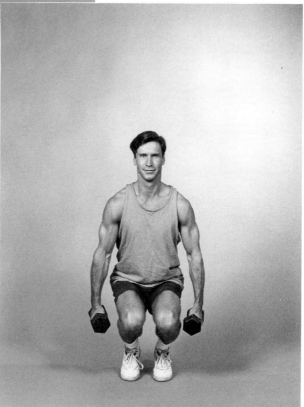

Finish

3 • Dumbbell Leg Curl

Develops, shapes, strengthens, and defines the hamstrings (back thigh) muscle.

Position: With a dumbbell placed between your feet, lie face down on a flat exercise bench or on the floor. Extend your legs straight out behind you and lean on your elbows for support.

Movement: Flexing your hamstrings (back thigh) muscles as you go, and keeping your feet together to hold the dumbbell in place, bending at the knees, raise your lower legs until they are perpendicular to the floor. Flex your hamstrings as hard as possible, and return to start position. Feel the stretch in your hamstrings and repeat the movement until you have completed your set.

Tips: Squeeze your knees together in order to help you flex your back thigh (hamstring) muscles on the upward movement. Do not jerk the weight up or nearly let it drop down to start position. Don't hold your breath. Breathe naturally.

Alternatives: This exercise can be done on any gym leg-curl machine.

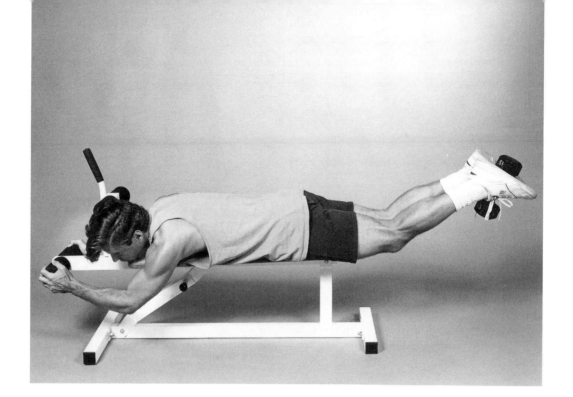

Start

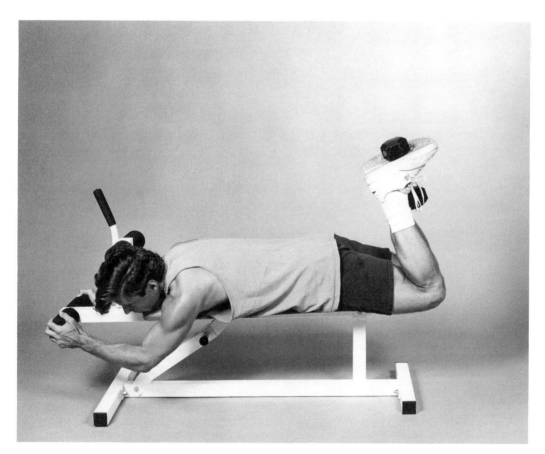

Finish

4 • Sissy Squat
(for Ironman and Superman workouts)

Develops, shapes, strengthens and defines the entire quadriceps (front thigh) muscle, especially the lower and inner area, and tightens and shapes the gluteus maximus (buttocks).

Position:	Stand with your feet a few inches apart and your toes pointed slightly outward. Place your hand on a stable object such as a post, high bench, or railing.
Movement:	Raise yourself up on your toes and, at the same time, lean your upper body back as far as you can (your buttocks will be nearly touching your heels) and feel a full stretch in your quadriceps muscles while at the same time flexing your buttocks muscles. You will be completely up on your toes at this point. Keep your hips in line with your ankles as you work. Flexing your quadriceps muscles as you go, return to start position and give your quadriceps muscles an extra hard flex. Repeat the movement until you have completed your set.
Tips:	The harder you flex, the more definition you will see.
Alternatives:	This exercise can be substituted for the standard leg extension.

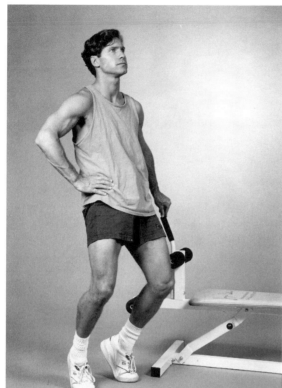

Start

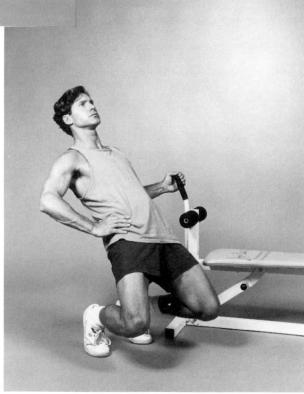

Finish

5 • Dumbbell Hack Squat
(for Superman workout)

Develops, shapes, defines, and strengthens the quadriceps (front thigh) muscle, especially the lower area, and helps to strengthen the hamstrings (back thigh) and gluteus maximus (buttocks) muscles.

Position: Stand with your feet a natural width apart and your toes pointed slightly outward, and hold a dumbbell in each hand, behind your back, palms facing away from your body and in line with each back thigh.

Movement: Bend at the knee into a squatting position, while at the same time letting the dumbbells descend in line with your back thighs. When you reach a position of thighs parallel to the floor, feel a full stretch in your quadriceps muscles. Flexing your quadriceps muscles as you go, return to start position. Give your quadriceps muscles an extra hard flex, and repeat the movement until you have completed your set.

Tips: If your anatomy allows it, go down a little lower on the low position. This will help give you greater definition.

Alternatives: You can perform this movement with a barbell held behind your back, or on any gym hack squat machine.

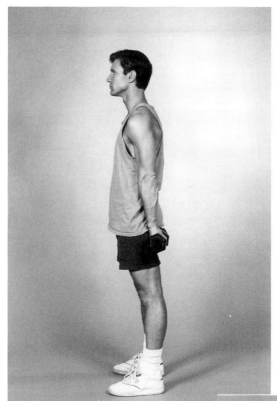

Start ——————————————————

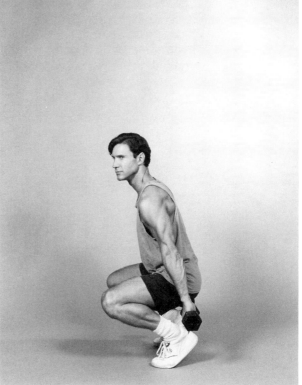

Finish ——————————————————

CALF ROUTINE

(Workout days two and four for those who choose the optional leg workout)

1 • Seated Straight-Toe Calf Raise

Develops, shapes, strengthens, and defines the entire calf muscle, especially the lower area.

Position: Sit at the edge of a flat exercise bench, with a dumbbell placed on each knee and your toes pointed straight ahead on a thick book or piece of wood. Lower your heels to the ground.

Movement: Flexing your calf muscles as you go, raise your toes as high as possible. Give your calves an extra flex on the up position and return to start, feeling a full stretch in your calf muscles. Repeat the movement until you have completed your set.

Tips: Keep your body stable. Do not rock back and forth. Don't hold your breath. Breathe naturally.

Alternatives: This exercise can be performed on any gym seated calf machine.

2 • Seated Angled-in-Toe Calf Raise

Develops, shapes, strengthens, and defines the entire calf muscle, especially the lower and outer area of this muscle.

Position and   Perform this exercise exactly as above, only angle your toes inward
Movement: as far as possible.

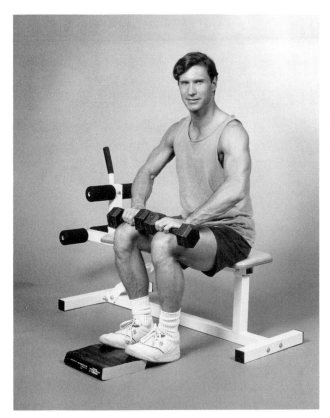

Seated Straight-Toe Calf Raise

Start

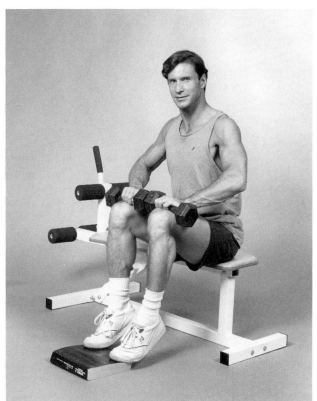

Seated Straight-Toe Calf Raise

Finish

143

3 • Standing Straight-Toe Calf Raise

Develops, shapes, strengthens, and defines the entire calf muscle.

Position: Stand near a holding object with a dumbbell in your left hand, and place the toes of your left foot at the edge of a thick book. Lower your heel as close to the ground as possible.

Movement: Flexing your left calf muscle as you go, raise yourself up onto your left toes until you cannot go any further. Flex your left calf muscle as hard as possible. Return to start position and feel a full stretch in your left calf muscle. Repeat the movement until you have completed your set. Then repeat the exercise for your other leg.

Tips: Rise fully up on your toes and descend completely down with each repetition. Don't cut the movements short.

Alternatives: You may perform this exercise at the edge of a stair, or on any standing gym calf machine.

4 • Standing Angled-out-Toe Calf Raise
(for Ironman and Superman workouts)

Develops, shapes, strengthens, and defines the entire calf muscle, especially the inner calf area.

Position and Movement: Perform this exercise exactly as above, only angle your toes as far outward as possible.

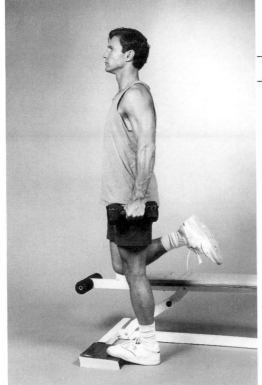

Standing Straight-Toe Calf Raise
Start

Standing Straight-Toe Calf Raise
Finish

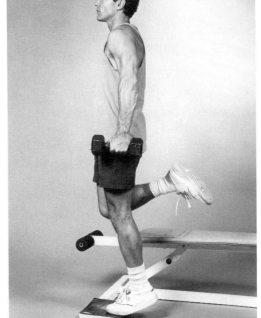

5 · Standing Angled-in-Toe Calf Raise
(for Superman workout)

Develops, shapes, strengthens, and defines the entire calf muscle, especially the outer calf area.

Position and Movement: Perform this exercise exactly as above, only angle your toes inward as far as possible.

REVIEW OF EXERCISES FOR EACH WORKOUT

THE FORTY-MINUTE, THREE-DAY-A-WEEK WORKOUT

Chest

1. Flat Dumbbell Press
2. Flat Dumbbell Flye
3. Incline Dumbbell Press
4. Incline Dumbbell Flye (Ironman and Superman)
5. Straight-Arm Cross-Bench Pullover (Superman)

Biceps

1. Seated Simultaneous Dumbbell Curl with a Twist
2. Seated Alternate Hammer Curl
3. Concentration Curl with a Twist
4. Lying Alternate Dumbbell Curl (Ironman and Superman)
5. Reverse Dumbbell Curl (Superman)

Triceps

1. Lying Dumbbell Extension
2. One-Arm Triceps Kickback with a Twist
3. Seated One-Arm Triceps Overhead Extension with a Twist
4. Cross-Face Triceps Extension (Ironman and Superman)
5. Dips Between Benches (Superman)

Abdominals

1. Alternate Knee-in
2. Knee-Raised Crunch
3. Squatting Side Bend
4. Reverse Crunch (Ironman and Superman)
5. Knee-Raised Twisting Sit-up (Superman)

Back

1. Double-Arm Bent Dumbbell Row
2. Single-Arm Bent Dumbbell Row
3. Upright Row
4. Dumbbell Deadlift Shrug (Ironman and Superman)
5. Seated Dumbbell Back Lateral (Superman)

Shoulders

1. Seated Simultaneous Dumbbell Press
2. Seated Side Lateral
3. Standing Bent Lateral with a Twist
4. Reverse Overhead Dumbbell Lateral (Ironman and Superman)
5. Pee-Wee Lateral (Superman)

SPLIT ROUTINE WORKOUT DAYS ONE AND THREE

Chest

1. Flat Dumbbell Press
2. Flat Dumbbell Flye
3. Incline Dumbbell Press
4. Incline Dumbbell Flye (Ironman and Superman)
5. Straight-Arm Cross-Bench Pullover (Superman)

Biceps

1. Seated Simultaneous Dumbbell Curl with a Twist
2. Seated Alternate Hammer Curl
3. Concentration Curl with a Twist
4. Lying Alternate Dumbbell Curl (Ironman and Superman)
5. Reverse Dumbbell Curl (Superman)

Triceps

1. Lying Dumbbell Extension
2. One-Arm Triceps Kickback with a Twist
3. Seated One-Arm Triceps Overhead Extension with a Twist
4. Cross-Face Triceps Extension (Ironman and Superman)
5. Dips Between Benches (Superman)

Abdominals

1. Alternate Knee-in
2. Knee-Raised Crunch
3. Squatting Side Bend
4. Reverse Crunch (Ironman and Superman)
5. Knee-Raised Twisting Sit-up (Superman)

SPLIT ROUTINE WORKOUT DAYS TWO AND FOUR

Abdominals

1. Alternate Knee-in
2. Knee-Raised Crunch
3. Squatting Side Bend
4. Reverse Crunch (Ironman and Superman)
5. Knee-Raised Twisting Sit-up (Superman)

Back

1. Double-Arm Bent Dumbbell Row
2. Single-Arm Bent Dumbbell Row
3. Upright Row
4. Dumbbell Deadlift Shrug (Ironman and Superman)
5. Seated Dumbbell Back Lateral (Superman)

Shoulders

1. Seated Simultaneous Dumbbell Press
2. Seated Side Lateral
3. Standing Bent Lateral with a Twist
4. Reverse Overhead Dumbbell Lateral (Ironman and Superman)
5. Pee-Wee Lateral (Superman)

Thighs (optional)

1. Regular Dumbbell Squat
2. Narrow Dumbbell Squat
3. Dumbbell Leg Curl
4. Sissy Squat (Ironman and Superman)
5. Dumbbell Hack Squat (Superman)

Calves (optional)

1. Seated Straight-Toe Calf Raise
2. Seated Angled-in-Toe Calf Raise
3. Standing Straight-Toe Calf Raise
4. Standing Angled-out-Toe Calf Raise (Ironman and Superman)
5. Standing Angled-in-Toe Calf Raise (Superman)

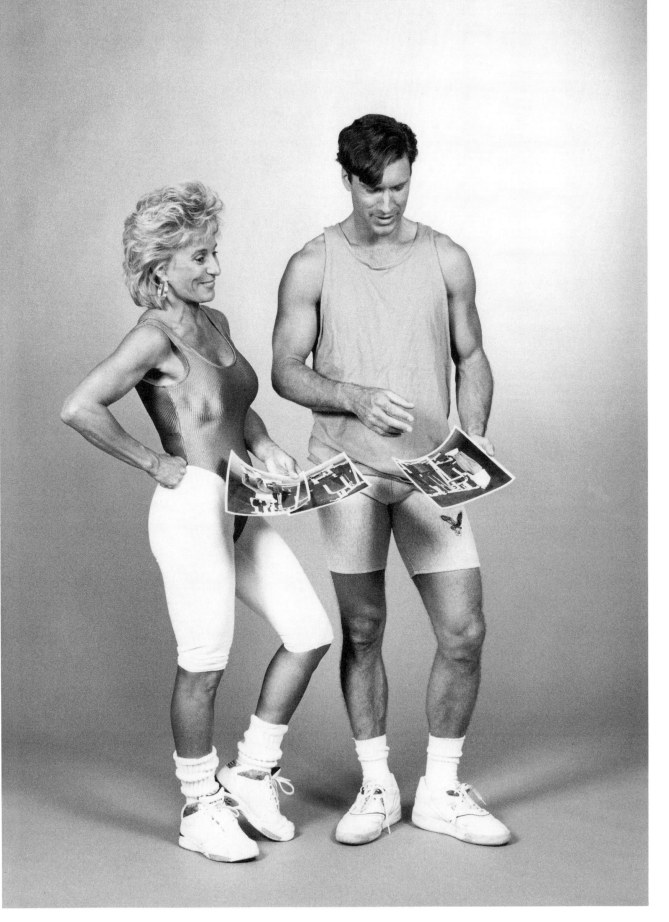

7

The Machine Workout

The exercises in this chapter can be done on either gym or home-gym machines. These days, there are virtually hundreds of different brands of machines, but when one takes a closer look, it becomes clear that the exercises performed on these machines require very similar stances and movements. The exercises in this chapter are demonstrated on my favorite home gym, the Health-trainer (see p. 241 for more information about this machine), but you can do them on any equivalent machine—either in a gym or at home.

Since some machines have different modes of operation, you will sometimes have to read the specific instructions for the gym machine you are using. (Most new gym machines have clearly written instruction cards.) In any case, you will find that the exercises are similar to the ones found in this chapter, and that you will have no trouble applying them to the machines you have at home or that are found in your fitness center.

For most body parts, two machine exercises are offered (for some body parts, three or four are offered). You can use all of the machine exercises, or you may pick and choose, using only the most important ones.

WHICH MACHINE EXERCISES ARE MOST IMPORTANT?

For your information, I have indicated which machine exercises are most important after each exercise title. These are the exercises used by champion bodybuilders on a regular basis. **They have an R next to them to indicate "regular basis."**

Other machine exercises are excellent as a change from free weights for the sake of variety. These exercises are used by champion bodybuilders as an option. **They have an O next to them to indicate "use as an option."**

If you love to work out with machines, and you find yourself using all of the machine exercises, both the R exercises and the O exercises, force yourself to eliminate the O exercises from time to time and replace them with the free weight exercises, so that you will achieve your best possible physique. (For a discussion on free weights versus machines, see p. 42.)

WORKOUT PLANS

This chapter contains the forty-minute, three-day plan, and the thirty-minute, four-day (or more) plan (the split routine). If you choose the split routine, you can exercise up to six days a week if you so desire, because the system allows for an automatic day of rest between body parts. If, however, you choose the three-day plan, you cannot work out more than three days a week, or you will violate the forty-eight-hour rest principle. (See pp. 4 and 43 for a review of this principle.)

THIRTY-MINUTE, THREE-DAY PLAN
(DO ON EACH WORKOUT DAY)

chest
biceps
triceps
abdominals
back
shoulders

SPLIT ROUTINE WORKOUT DAYS ONE AND THREE	SPLIT ROUTINE WORKOUT DAYS TWO AND FOUR
chest	abdominals
biceps	back
triceps	shoulders
abdominals	thighs (optional)
	calves (optional)

If you choose to exercise your legs, you will have to use the split routine because it is too much work to exercise eight body parts in one day. Reminders of when to stop exercising if you are on the forty-minute, three-day workout, or a split routine will be given in the exercise instructions, and reviewed at the end of the chapter.

This chapter will also include the optional Ironman and Superman routines that ask you to add one or two exercises to each body part. If you are doing either of these routines, since you will be adding time to your workout, you may want to do a split routine, but if you have the energy, of course you can do the workout all in one day. (A discussion of the Superman and Ironman workouts is found on p. 58.)

A WORD ABOUT WEIGHTS

The exercise instructions will include a section for suggested beginning weights. Don't feel obligated to stick to those prescriptions. Since you have the option of using such a wide variety of weights (you don't have to go out and buy them—they come with the machine), test the weights for yourself.

If you can get twelve strict repetitions for your first set without straining, and yet without feeling that you could have gotten a lot more repetitions; and, if you can get ten repetitions for your second set at the higher weight without a big struggle, yet without feeling that you could have done another five or six repetitions; and, if you can get six to eight strict repetitions for your last set without killing yourself, and also without feeling that you could have gotten a few more reps, those are your correct beginning weights.

Sometimes you will find that my suggested beginning weight is too light. Other times, you will find that my suggested beginning weight is too heavy. It's up to you to see what is best for you. However, if you are in doubt as to which weight to use, in the beginning stages of your workout it is much better to go too light than to go too heavy, because at this stage, the most important thing is to learn to do the exercises in strict form, and you will not be able to do this if you are struggling with too-heavy weights.

You will also note that the weights used on the machines are somewhat higher than the weights used in the dumbbell workout. This is due to the physics involved in machine weight lifting. More weight is needed to make up for the mechanical operation of the machine. In other words, you will notice that you can do a double-arm cable curl of sixty pounds using the same amount of strength it would take you to do a double-arm cable curl with two fifteen-pound dumbbells—(thirty pounds in all, half the weight).

The half-weight rule does not always apply, because each machine has different "physics." The best thing you can do for yourself when working with machines is to resist false comparisons between the heaviness of your dumbbells and the heaviness of the machine weights. There is simply no equation, except to say that with a machine you will always have to use a heavier weight in order to equal the weight of the dumbbells.

CHEST ROUTINE

1 • Seated Machine Press (O)

Increases strength and mass of the entire pectoral (chest) muscle.

Position: Sit in the seat of the machine press station with your feet flat on the floor and your hands gripping the pressing bar at the lower handles.

Movement: Using the strength of your pectoral muscles and not your arms, and flexing your pectoral muscles as you go, press the bar forward until your arms are fully extended. Give your pectoral muscles an extra hard flex, and return to start position. Feel the stretch in your chest muscles, and repeat the movement until you have completed your set.

Tips: Don't jerk the bar forward or nearly let it drop back into place. Control the weights at all times. Do not let the plates make contact on the return movement.

Weights: Fifty, sixty, and seventy pounds. Increase overall weights as you get stronger.

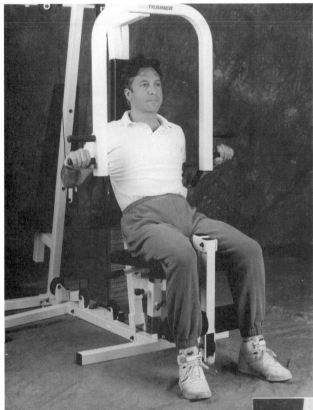

Start ———————————————

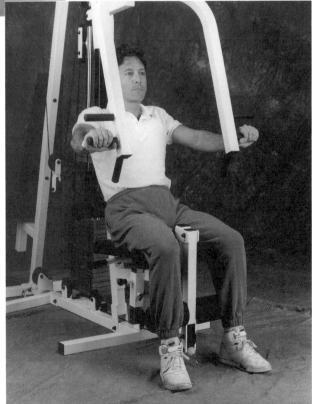

Finish ————————————

155

2 • Pec-Deck Machine (R)

Develops, shapes, defines, and strengthens the entire pectoral (chest) muscle.

Position: Sit at the seat of the pec-deck machine. Grip the upper end of the pad itself, and place your forearms on the pads so that they run down the full length of the pads.

Movement: Using your pectoral muscles only, and flexing those muscles as you go, move the pads forward until you cannot go any further. Give your pectoral muscles an extra flex, and in full control, return to start position. Allow the machine to stretch out your pectoral muscles by letting your arms extend slightly backward. Repeat the movement until you have completed your set.

Tips: Beware of the temptation to jerk the weights forward and to nearly let them drop back to position. Use controlled, deliberate movements. Don't allow the weight plates to touch on the return movement. Don't hold your breath. Breathe naturally.

Weights: Forty, fifty, and sixty pounds. Increase overall weights as you get stronger.

3 • Incline Dumbbell Press
(Follow the instructions on p. 78.)

4 • Incline Dumbell Flye
(For Ironman and Superman workouts)
(Follow the instructions on p. 79.)

5 • Straight-Arm Cross-Bench Pullover
(For Superman workout)
(Follow the instructions on pp. 80–81.)

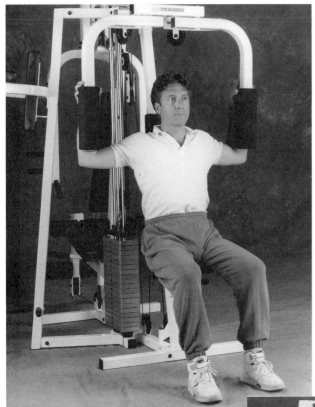

Pec-Deck Machine
Start ————————————

Pec-Deck Machine
Finish ——————————

BICEPS ROUTINE

1 • Double-Arm Cable Curl (O)

Develops, shapes, strengthens, and defines the entire biceps muscle, especially the peak of the muscle.

Position: Attach a short bar to the floor cable. Stand with your feet a natural width apart and grip the bar with an underhand grip, holding the bar so that your hands are about two inches from the end of the bar. Extend your arms fully downward.

Movement: Keeping your elbows riveted to your upper body, and flexing your biceps as you go, curl the bar upward until you cannot go any further. Give your biceps an extra flex, and in full control, return to start position. Feel the stretch in your biceps muscles and repeat the movement until you have completed your set.

Tips: Do not jerk the bar upward or nearly let it drop down to start position. Maintain full control of the movement at all times. Don't let your elbows wander away from your body.

Weights: Fifty, sixty, and seventy pounds. Increase overall weights as you get stronger.

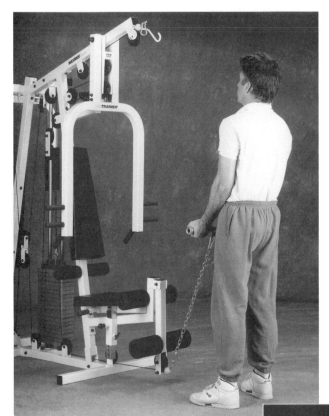

Start ————————————

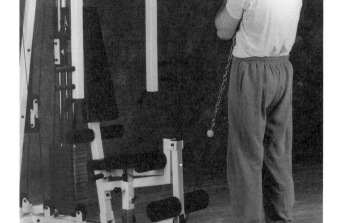

Finish ——————

2 • Machine Biceps Pulldown (O)

Develops, shapes, strengthens, and defines the entire biceps muscle.

Position: Place a short bar on the lat-pulldown machine. Grip the bar with palms facing your body, and sit in the machine seat, letting your arms fully extend upward.

Movement: Keeping your arms close to your body, and using the strength of your biceps muscles only, and flexing your biceps muscles as you go, pull the bar down until your elbows can descend no further. Give your biceps muscles an extra hard flex, and return to start position. Feel the stretch in your biceps muscles and repeat the movement until you have completed your set.

Tips: Do not let your elbows wander away from your body throughout the movement. Do not jerk the bar down or nearly let it fly up to start position. Maintain control at all times.

Weights: Fifty, sixty, and seventy pounds. Increase overall weights as you get stronger.

3 • Concentration Curl with a Twist
(Follow the instructions on pp. 86–87.)

4 • Lying Alternate Dumbbell Curl
(For Ironman and Superman workouts)
(Follow the instructions on pp. 88–89.)

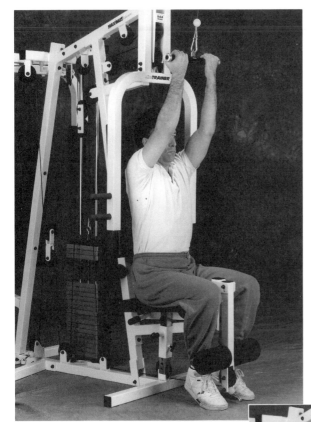

Machine Biceps Pulldown

Start ———————————

Machine Biceps Pulldown

Finish ————————

5 • Reverse Machine Curl (O)
(For Superman workout)

Develops, strengthens, shapes, and defines the entire biceps muscle, especially the outer area, and helps to build the forearm.

Position: Attach a short bar to the floor cable. Stand with your feet a natural width apart and grip the bar with an overhand grip, holding the bar so that your hands are about two inches from the end of the bar. Extend your arms fully downward.

Movement: Keeping your elbows riveted to your upper body, flexing your biceps as you go, curl the bar upward until you cannot go any further. Give your biceps an extra flex, and in full control, return to start position. Feel the stretch in your biceps muscles, and repeat the movement until you have completed your set.

Tips: Do not swing the bar upward. Keep your elbows close to your body. Don't hold your breath. Breathe naturally.

Weights: Fifty, sixty, and seventy pounds. Increase overall weights as you get stronger.

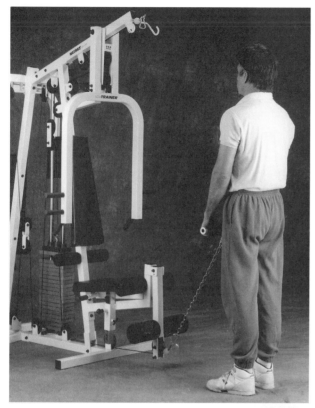

Start ———————————————

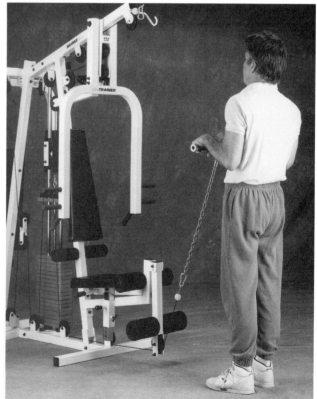

Finish ————————————

TRICEPS ROUTINE

1 • Triceps Pushdown (R)

Develops, shapes, strengthens, and defines the entire triceps muscle.

Position: Place the short bar on the lat-pulldown machine and grasp the bar with an overhand grip. Bend at the elbows and fully extend your forearms upward. Rivet your upper arms to your body (don't let your elbows wander away from your body throughout the movement). Stand erect.

Movement: Using only the strength of your triceps muscles, and flexing those muscles as you go, press the bar down until you cannot go any further, and your elbows are nearly locked. Give your triceps muscles an extra hard flex, and in full control, return to start position, letting the bar come up as high as possible, and feeling the stretch in your triceps muscles. Repeat the movement until you have completed your set.

Tips: Do not lean forward in an effort to help yourself in pushing down the weight. If the weight is too heavy, go lighter. Perform each repetition in strict, controlled form.

Weights: Fifty, sixty, and seventy pounds. Increase overall weights as you get stronger.

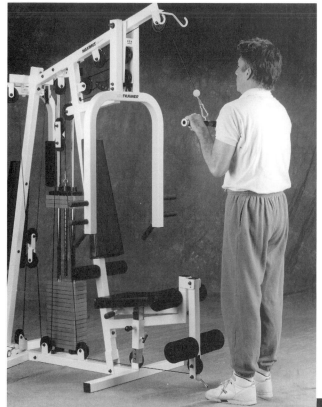

Start ————————————

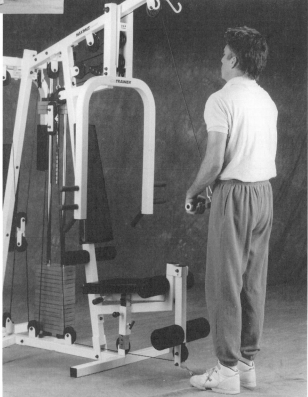

Finish ——————————

2 • Pulley Triceps Kickback (O)

Develops, shapes, strengthens, and defines the entire triceps muscle, especially the upper area.

Position: Attach the triangular or overhand "D" handle device to the lower pulley. Grip the handle with an overhand grip (palm facing up). Bend at the waist so that your back is nearly parallel to the floor and bend at the elbow (you could be looking at your fist).

Movement: Keeping your upper arm close to your body, and using the strength of your triceps muscle only, and flexing that muscle as you go, extend your working arm straight out behind you until your elbow is nearly locked. Give your triceps muscle an extra flex and return to start position. Feel the stretch in your triceps muscle, and repeat the movement until you have completed your set. Repeat the set for your other arm.

Tips: Don't let your elbow wander away from your body.

Weights: Thirty, forty, and fifty pounds. Increase overall weights as you get stronger.

3 • Seated One-Arm Triceps Overhead Extension with a Twist
(Follow the instructions on pp. 96–97.)

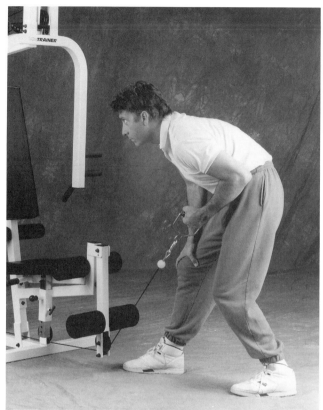

Pulley Triceps Kickback
Start —————————————

Pulley Triceps Kickback
Finish —————————————

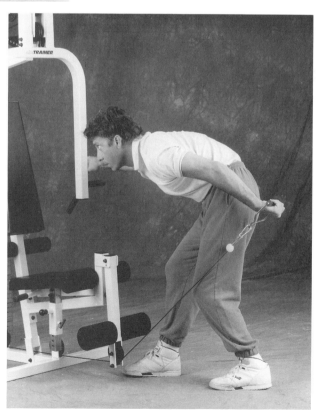

4 • Overhead Triceps Extension (R)
(For Ironman and Superman workouts)

Develops, shapes, strengthens, and defines the entire triceps muscle.

Position:	Attach the short, straight, or a curved triceps bar to the high pulley. Facing away from the machine, place one foot about fifteen inches in front of the other, and grasp the bar at either end with an overhand grip (palms facing away from your body). Bend fully at the elbows, with your upper arms close to your head.
Movement:	In a smooth, controlled motion, and using only the strength of your triceps muscles, and flexing your triceps muscles as you go, extend your arms outward until your elbows are locked. Give your triceps muscles an extra flex, and return to start position. Let the weights stretch out your triceps muscles and repeat the movement until you have completed your set.
Tips:	Don't jerk the bar forward or nearly let it drop back to start position. Do not hold your breath. Breathe naturally.
Weights:	Thirty, forty, and fifty pounds. Increase overall weights as you get stronger.

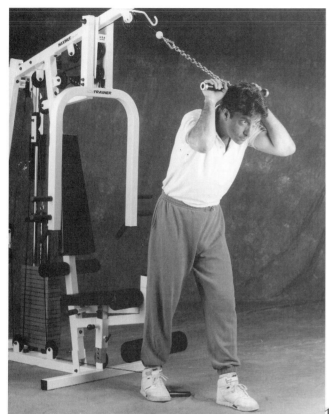

Start

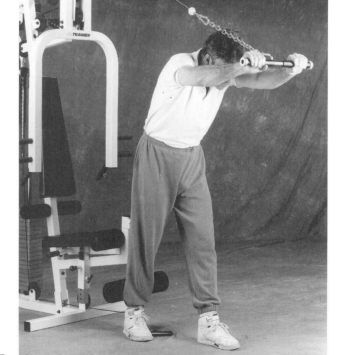

Finish

5 • High Bar Dip (O)
(For Superman workout)

Develops, shapes, strengthens, and defines the entire triceps muscle, especially the elbow area, and adds thickness to the muscle.

Position: Facing the machine, grasp the dip handles, palms facing downward, and jump up to a support position with your arms straight and your elbows locked.

Movement: Keeping your elbows close to your body as you go, and bending at the elbows, in a smooth and controlled movement slowly lower your body until you cannot go any further. Feel a full stretch in your triceps muscles. Using the strength of your triceps muscles, return to start position, and give your triceps muscles an extra hard flex. Repeat the movement until you have completed your set.

Tips: Don't lurch yourself upward or nearly drop down to the low position. Maintain a fluid movement.

Weights: You will not use weights for this exercise.

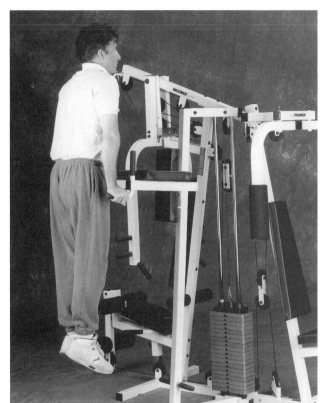

Start

Finish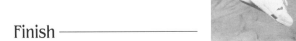

ABDOMINAL ROUTINE

1 • Machine Crunch (O)

Develops, shapes, strengthens, and defines the upper abdominal muscles, and helps to develop the lower abdominal area.

Position: Place the short bar on the lat-pulldown machine. Sit at the seat of the pulldown machine, your back to the machine. Bend at the elbows and grip the bar at each end, palms facing your body. Your back should be straight and your head erect.

Movement: In one fluid movement, crunch your upper body down until your elbows nearly touch your knee-thigh area—but while you're crunching, flex your upper abdominal muscles as hard as possible. Keeping the pressure on your upper abdominal muscles, return to start position and repeat the movement until you have completed your set.

Tips: Do not pull the bar with arm strength. Use your arms as a lever. Use abdominal strength to pull the bar.

Weights: Twenty, thirty, and forty pounds.

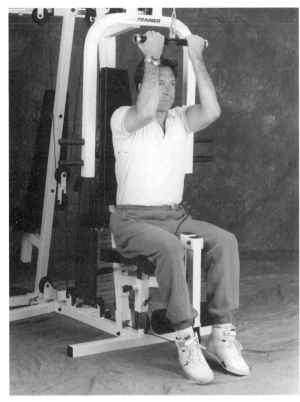

Start ————————————

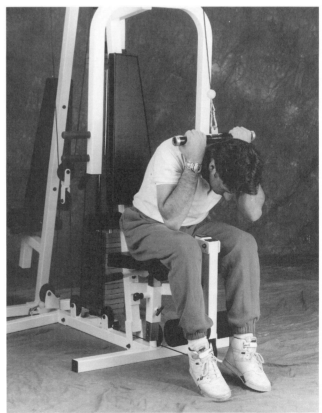

Finish ————————————

2 • Knee-Raised Crunch
(Follow the instructions on pp. 104–5.)

3 • Squatting Side Bend
(Follow the instructions on pp. 106–7.)

4 • Reverse Crunch
(for Ironman and Superman workouts)

(Follow the instructions on pp. 108–109.)

---

5 • Knee-Raised Twisting Sit-up
(for Superman workout)

(Follow the instructions on pp. 110–111.)

Note: If you are following a split routine, stop here. Your workout days one and three are over. If you are following a three-day-a-week plan, continue on and do your back and shoulders.

BACK ROUTINE

1 • Lat Pulldown to the Front (R)

Develops, shapes, strengthens, and defines the latissimus dorsi muscles, especially the upper area.

Position: Sit at the seat of the lat-pulldown machine so that your ankles fit snugly under the ankle pads, and grasp and lat-pulldown bar as wide as possible. Your palms should be facing away from your body.

Movement: Flexing your latissimus dorsi muscles as you go, pull the bar down until it touches your upper chest. Give your lat muscles an extra hard flex and return to start position, until your arms are fully extended upward, and you can feel a full stretch in your latissimus dorsi muscles. Repeat the movement until you have completed your set.

Tips: Keep your body steady. Do not rock back and forth. Be sure that it is your lat muscles, and not your arms, that are doing the work.

Weights: Fifty, sixty, and seventy pounds. Increase overall weights as you get stronger.

2 • Narrow-Grip Lat Pulldown to the Front (R)

Develops, shapes, strengthens, and defines the latissimus dorsi muscles, especially the lower area.

Position and Movement: Perform this exercise exactly as you perform the lat pulldown to the front, only use the narrow bar with handles, or grip the regular lat-pulldown bar with hands placed no wider apart than the width of your chest.

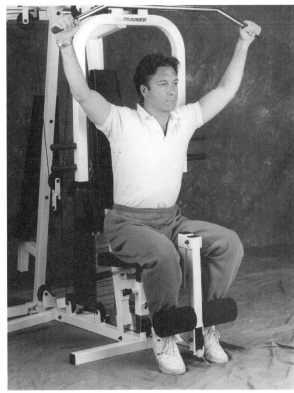

Lat Pulldown to Front
Start ————————————————

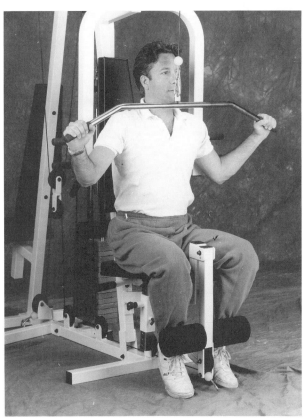

Lat Pulldown to Front
Finish ————————————————

3 • Machine Upright Row (O)

Develops, shapes, strengthens, and defines the trapezius muscles. Also helps to develop the front deltoid (shoulder) muscles.

Position: Attach a narrow bar to the floor pulley. Stand with your feet a natural width apart, facing the machine, and grip the bar with an overhand grip, hands about six to eight inches apart (palms facing your body), and your arms fully extended downward. The bar should be centered in front of your thighs.

Movement: Keeping the bar close to your body throughout the movement, and flexing your trapezius muscles as you go, pull the bar upward, letting the bar graze your stomach and chest as you go—until the bar reaches chin height. (Your elbows will be fully extended outward at this point.) Give your trapezius muscles an extra hard flex, and in full control, return to start position. Feel the stretch in your trapezius muscles. Repeat the movement until you have completed your set.

Tips: Do not jerk the bar upward or nearly let it drop down to start position. Maintain full control at all times. Don't bend your back in an effort to make the work easier. If the weight is too heavy to allow you to perform strict repetitions, decrease the weight.

Weights: Forty, fifty, and sixty pounds. Increase overall weights as you get stronger.

4 • Dumbbell Deadlift Shrug
(for Ironman and Superman workouts)
(Follow the instructions on pp. 118–119.)

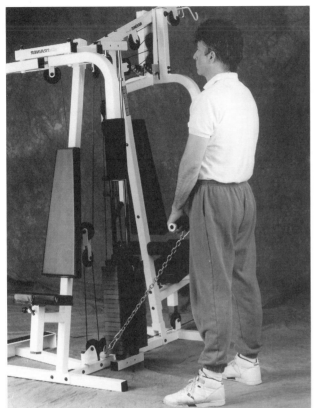

Machine Upright Row

Start

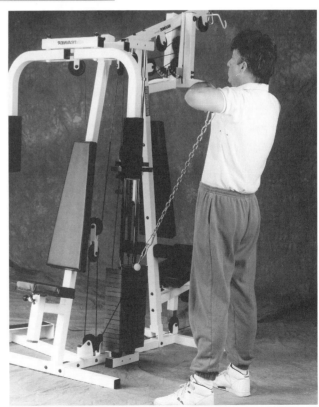

Machine Upright Row

Finish

5 • Seated Cable Pulley Row (R)
(for Superman workout)

Develops, thickens, and strengthens the entire back, especially the lower latissimus dorsi area.

Position: Attach the rowing handles or a short bar to the low pulley, and take hold of the handles or bar, palms facing your body. Bend at the knees and place your feet against the frame of the machine, or on the metal footrest. Extend your arms fully and lean forward, letting the weights stretch out your back. Be sure that your body is far enough from the weights so that when you stretch fully forward, the plates do not touch.

Movement: Keeping your back straight, and bending at the elbows and flexing your back muscles as you go, and keeping your elbows close to your body, pull the handles toward your waist until the bar touches your upper waist area. You should end up in a nearly perpendicular position. Give your back muscles an extra hard flex, and return to start position. Feel a full stretch in your back muscles, and repeat the movement until you have completed your set.

Tips: Arch your back and push out your chest at the end of each movement. Be sure that you are sitting upright at the end of each movement, rather than leaning forward or backward. Beware of the temptation to start pulling with your arms. Force your back muscles to do the work. Don't rock forward and backward in an effort to make the work easier.

Weights: Forty, fifty, and sixty pounds. Increase overall weights as you get stronger.

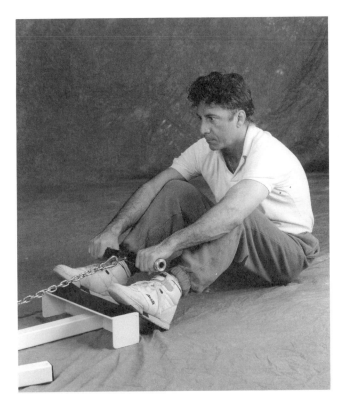

Start

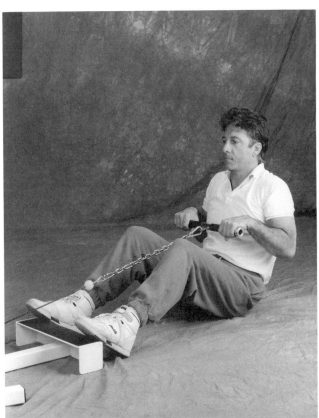

Finish

SHOULDERS

1 • Machine Shoulder Press (O)

Develops, strengthens, shapes, and defines the entire deltoid (shoulder) muscle, especially the front area.

Position: Sit in the seat of the shoulder pressing device (this is the same seat as used for seated machine press for chest). Set the bar to maximum forward position. Grasp the pressing bar at the very bottom, gripping the lower horizontal handles, palms facing away from your body. Lean forward.

Movement: Keeping your chest out and your back straight, and flexing your shoulder muscles as you go, press the bar upward and out, using only shoulder strength, until your arms are fully extended out in front of you. Give your shoulder muscles an extra hard flex, and return to start position. Feel a full stretch in your shoulder muscles and repeat the movement until you have completed your set.

Tips: Do not jerk the bar forward or nearly let it drop back to start position. Maintain control at all times. Do not hold your breath. Breathe naturally.

Weights: Forty, fifty, and sixty pounds. Increase overall weights as you get stronger.

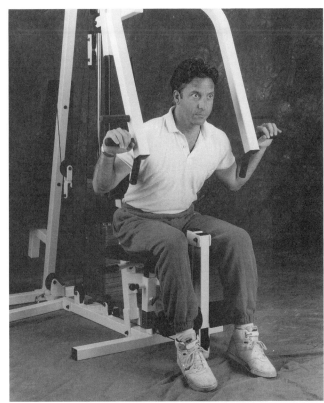

Start —————————————

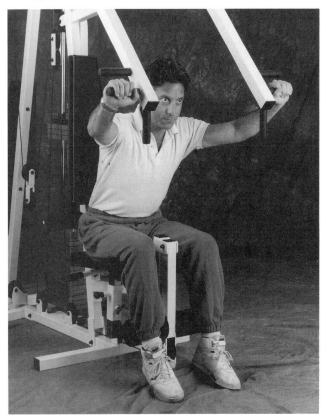

Finish —————————————

2 • Bent-Over Cable Side Lateral Raise (O)

Develops, shapes, strengthens, and defines the entire deltoid (shoulder) muscle, especially the side area.

Position: Attach a triangle handle or "D" handle to the floor pulley and grasp the handle with one hand, in an overhand grip. Stand sideways toward the machine. Extend the gripping hand fully downward.

Movement: Bend at the waist, and flexing your shoulder muscle as you go, rotate your arm and shoulder up and out until your arm is nearly parallel to your shoulders. Give your shoulder muscle an extra hard flex, and return to start position. Feel a full stretch in your shoulder muscle and repeat the movement until you have completed your set. Repeat the set for your other arm.

Tips: Keep your arm close to your body throughout the movement. Do not jerk the cable back or nearly let it drop down to start position. Maintain control at all times. Do not hold your breath. Breathe naturally.

Weights: Forty, fifty, and sixty pounds. Increase overall weights as you get stronger.

3 • Standing Bent Lateral with a Twist
(Follow the instructions on pp. 126–127.)

4 • Reverse Overhead Dumbbell Lateral
(for Ironman and Superman workouts)
(Follow the instructions on pp. 128–129.)

5 • Pee-Wee Lateral
(for Superman workout)
(Follow the instructions on pp. 130–131.)

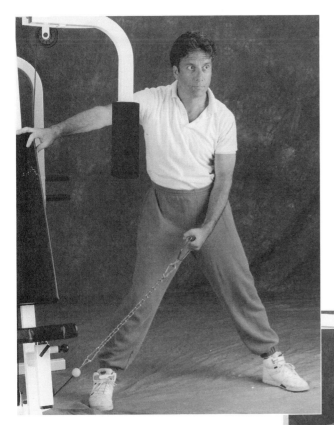

Bent-Over Cable Side Lateral Raise

Start ———————————————————

Bent-Over Cable Side Lateral Raise

Finish ———————————————

Stop: If you are doing a three-day routine, your workout is completed. Congratulations.

Go: If you are doing a split routine, you must now exercise your abdominals for workout days two and four and if in addition you are doing the optional leg workout, you must now proceed to do the thigh and calf routines.

THIGH ROUTINE

(Workout days two and four for those who choose the optional leg workout)

1 • Regular Dumbbell Squat

(Follow the instructions on pp. 132–133.)

2 • Narrow Dumbbell Squat

(Follow the instructions on pp. 134–135.)

3 • Standing Leg Curl (R)

Develops, shapes, strengthens, and defines the hamstrings (back thigh) muscles.

Position: Face the pressing bar, and adjust the seat height so that the seat is at the lowest position. Grasp the pressing bar for support, and lean slightly forward. Place your left calf behind the roller pad—with your toes nearly touching the machine base.

Movement: Flexing your left hamstrings (back thigh muscles) as you go, bending at the knee, curl your left leg up, bringing your right heel toward your left buttocks—until you cannot go any further. Give your hamstrings an extra hard flex, and in full control, return to start position. Feel the stretch in your left back thigh muscle, and repeat the movement until you have completed your set. Repeat the set for your right leg.

Tips: Do not jerk the weights up, or nearly let them drop down to place. Maintain control at all times. Do not move from side to side. Keep your upper body steady.

Weights: Thirty, forty, and fifty pounds. Increase overall weights as you get stronger.

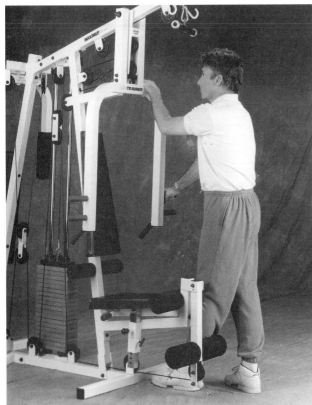

Standing Leg Curl
Start

Standing Leg Curl
Finish

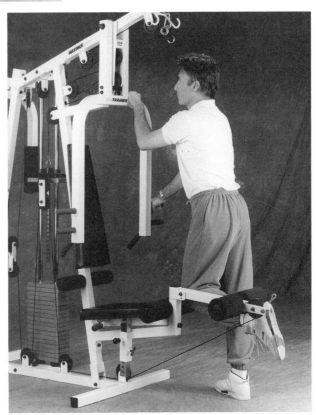

4 · Leg Extension (R)
(for Ironman and Superman workouts)

Defines, shapes, and develops the quadriceps (front thigh) muscle, and develops and strengthens the knee area. (This exercise is often prescribed by doctors as healing therapy for knee injuries.)

Position: Sit in the seat of the leg extension machine, and place your insteps under the roller pads. Place your back flat against the seat back, and grasp the side holding bars or the side edges of the seat.

Movement: Flexing your quadriceps (front thigh) muscles as you go, extend your legs outward until you cannot go any further, and your legs are straight out in front of you. Give your quadriceps muscles an extra hard flex. Return to start position and feel the stretch in your quadriceps muscles. Repeat the movement until you have completed your set.

Tips: Do not lift your buttocks off the seat and/or lean forward in an effort to jerk the weight up in order to make the work easier.

Weights: Forty, fifty, and sixty pounds. Increase overall weights as you get stronger.

5 · Dumbbell Hack Squat
(for Superman workout)
(Follow the instructions on pp. 140–141.)

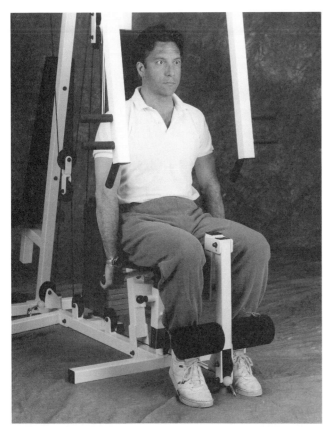

Leg Extension
Start

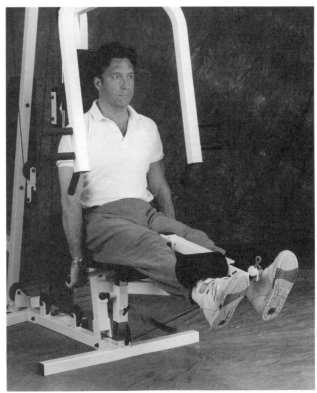

Leg Extension
Finish

CALF ROUTINE

1 • Standing Straight-Toe Machine Calf Raise (R)

Develops, shapes, strengthens, and defines the entire calf muscle, especially the lower area.

Position: Place the short bar on the lower pulley. Stand on the four-inch by four-inch steel foot plate, facing the machine, and with the soles of your feet centered at the edge of the foot plate. Your heels should be as low to the floor as possible. Hold on to the pulley in an overhand grip (palms facing your body).

Movement: Flexing your calf muscles as you go, raise your heels and stand on the tips of your toes until you cannot go any further. (You will be automatically pulling up the stack of weights.) Give your calf muscles an extra hard flex and return to start position.

Tips: Do not jerk yourself up to finish position, or nearly drop down to start. Maintain control at all times.

Weights: Seventy, eighty, and ninety pounds. Increase overall weights as you get stronger.

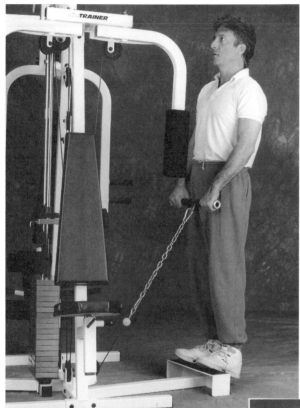

Standing Straight-Toe Machine Calf Raise

Start

Standing Straight-Toe Machine Calf Raise

Finish

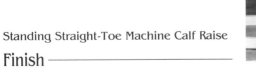

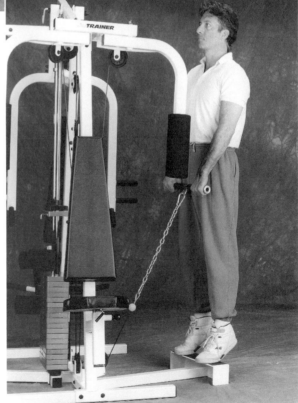

2 • Standing Angled-out-Toe Machine Calf Raise (O)

Develops, strengthens, shapes, and defines the entire calf muscle, especially the inner area.

Position and Movement: Follow the instructions for the standing straight-toe machine calf raise (p. 190), only angle your toes out as far as possible throughout the exercises.

3 • Standing Angled-in-Toe Machine Calf Raise (O)

Develops, strengthens, shapes, and defines the entire calf muscle, especially the outer area.

Position and Movement: Follow the instructions for the standing straight-toe machine calf raise (p. 190), only angle your toes in as far as possible.

4 • Seated Straight-Toe Calf Raise
(for Ironman and Superman workouts)
(Follow the instructions on pp. 142–143.)

5 • Seated Angled-in-Toe Calf Raise
(for Superman workout)
(Follow the instructions on p. 142.)

REVIEW OF EXERCISES FOR EACH WORKOUT

THE FORTY-MINUTE, THREE-DAY-A-WEEK WORKOUT

Chest

1. Seated Machine Press (O)
2. Pec-Deck Machine (R)
3. Incline Dumbell Press
4. Incline Dumbbell Flye (Ironman and Superman)
5. Straight-Arm Cross-Bench Pullover (Superman)

Biceps

1. Double-Arm Cable Curl (O)
2. Machine Biceps Pulldown (O)
3. Concentration Curl with a Twist
4. Lying Alternate Dumbbell Curl (Ironman and Superman)
5. Reverse Machine Curl (O) (Superman)

Triceps

1. Triceps Pushdown (R)
2. Pulley Triceps Kickback (O)
3. Seated One-Arm Triceps Overhead Extension with a Twist
4. Overhead Triceps Extension (R) (Ironman and Superman)
5. High Bar Dip (O) (Superman)

Abdominals

1. Machine Crunch (O)
2. Knee-Raised Crunch
3. Squatting Side Bend
4. Reverse Crunch (Ironman and Superman)
5. Knee-Raised Twisting Sit-up (Superman)

Back

1. Lat Pulldown to the Front (R)
2. Narrow-Grip Lat Pulldown to the Front (R)
3. Machine Upright Row (O)
4. Dumbbell Deadlift Shrug (Ironman and Superman)
5. Seated Cable Pulley Row (R) (Superman)

Shoulders

1. Machine Shoulder Press (O)
2. Bent-Over Cable Side Lateral Raise (O)
3. Standing Bent Lateral with a Twist
4. Reverse Overhead Dumbbell Lateral (Ironman and Superman)
5. Pee-Wee Lateral (Superman)

THE SPLIT ROUTINE WORKOUT DAYS ONE AND THREE

Chest

1. Seated Machine Press (O)
2. Pec-Deck Machine (R)
3. Incline Dumbell Press
4. Incline Dumbbell Flye (Ironman and Superman)
5. Straight-Arm Cross-Bench Pullover (Superman)

Biceps

1. Double-Arm Cable Curl (O)
2. Machine Biceps Pulldown (O)
3. Concentration Curl with a Twist
4. Lying Alternate Dumbbell Curl (Ironman and Superman)
5. Reverse Machine Curl (O) (Superman)

Triceps

1. Triceps Pushdown (R)
2. Pulley Triceps Kickback (O)
3. Seated One-Arm Triceps Overhead Extension with a Twist
4. Overhead Triceps Extension (R) (Ironman and Superman)
5. High Bar Dip (O) (Superman)

Abdominals

1. Machine Crunch (O)
2. Knee-Raised Crunch
3. Squatting Side Bend
4. Reverse Crunch (Ironman and Superman)
5. Knee-Raised Twisting Sit-up (Superman)

SPLIT ROUTINE WORKOUT DAYS TWO AND FOUR

Abdominals

1. Machine Crunch (O)
2. Knee-Raised Crunch
3. Squatting Side Bend
4. Reverse Crunch (Ironman and Superman)
5. Knee-Raised Twisting Sit-up (Superman)

Back

1. Lat Pulldown to the Front (R)
2. Narrow-Grip Lat Pulldown to the Front (R)
3. Machine Upright Row (O)
4. Dumbbell Deadlift Shrug (Ironman and Superman)
5. Seated Cable Pulley Row (R) (Superman)

Shoulders

1. Machine Shoulder Press (O)
3. Bent-Over Cable Side Lateral Raise (O)
3. Standing Bent Lateral with a Twist
4. Reverse Overhead Dumbbell Lateral (Ironman and Superman)
5. Pee-Wee Lateral (Superman)

Thighs (optional)

1. Regular Dumbbell Squat
2. Narrow Dumbbell Squat
3. Standing Leg Curl (R)
4. Leg Extension (R) (Ironman and Superman)
5. Dumbbell Hack Squat (Superman)

Calves (optional)

1. Standing Straight-Toe Machine Calf Raise (R)
2. Standing Angled-out-Toe Machine Calf Raise (O)
3. Standing Angled-in-Toe Machine Calf Raise (O)
4. Seated Straight-Toe Calf Raise (Ironman and Superman)
5. Seated Angled-in-Toe Calf Raise (Superman)

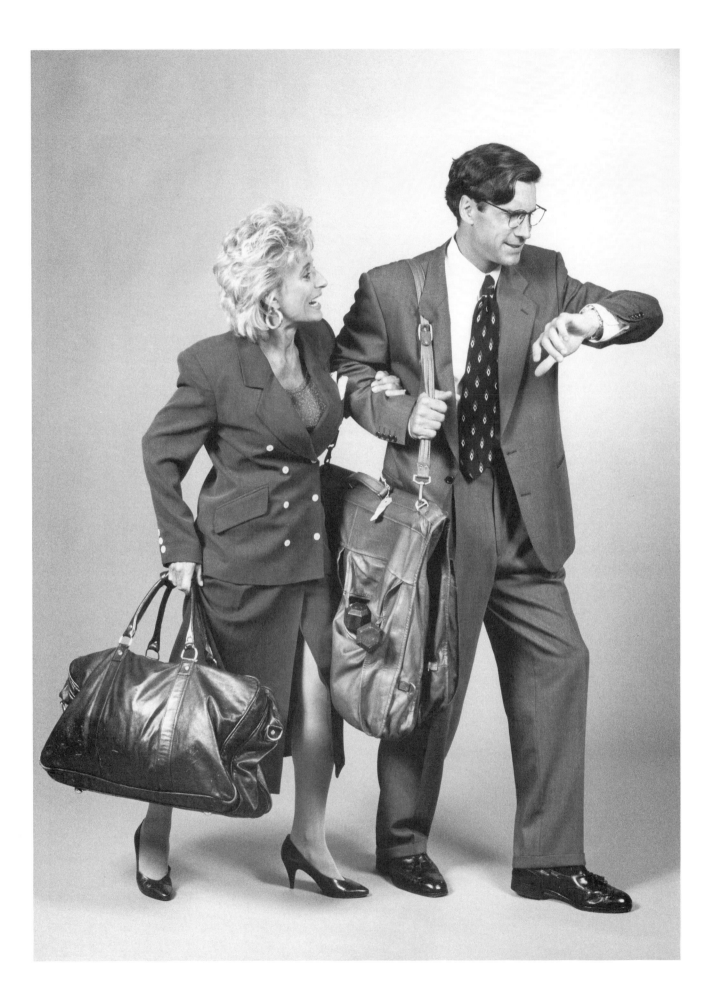

8

On the Road

Once you start a workout, and are into it for some time, it's a real threat to think that if you are away from home you'll have to stop working out— and that you will lose the hard-earned ground you have gained. Well, there's good news. No matter where you travel in the world—whether you go on a business trip or a vacation, there is a way for you to work out, and to eat, so that you do not have to lose ground. First we'll discuss the workout, then the eating plan.

Workout conditions vary. If you are a businessman, you may stay in hotels with sparsely equipped gyms. But what if you get a hotel that has no gym at all? Is there something you can do in your room? Of course there is. First we'll talk about sparsely equipped hotel gyms of every kind, and then we'll talk about what you can do in your room.

Finally, we'll discuss ways to keep up your low-fat eating plan (Chapter 9), even in the most difficult situations.

SPARSELY EQUIPPED HOTEL GYMS

Fortunately, these days many hotels offer gyms that are not sparsely equipped, and in fact have equipment equal to or better than the equipment found in your local fitness center or home gym. If this is the case, no problem. Simply follow the workout contained in Chapter 6 or 7. But what should you do in other situations. Let's look at several possible scenarios.

One Total-Body Exercise Machine but No Free Weights

If the gym offers a machine, such as the one described in Chapter 7, but no free weights, obviously you'll have to forget free weights for the short time that you are using that gym. Don't worry. Your body will not lose ground if you don't work out the ideal way (that is, with a generous amount of free weight exercises) for a while.

If the machine is a good, overall total-body workout machine, and is equivalent to the one used in Chapter 7, do all of the machine exercises prescribed in that chapter. This will mean that you will have done at least two exercises per body part, and three or four exercises for some body parts.

What should you do to make up for the required third exercise per body part (and the fourth or fifth exercise, if you are following the Ironman or Superman workout)? Since there are no free weights, you'll have to double up on some of the machine exercises.

For example, if the hotel gym machine offers only two possible exercises for the chest—the seated machine press and the pec-deck exercise, and you are doing the regular workout, do your three sets for the seated machine press exercise, and then do your three sets for the pec-deck exercise, and then go back to the seated machine press and do another three sets of that exercise. This will give you the equivalent of three chest exercises—or nine total sets—the required amount for the the regular Top Shape Workout.

If you are doing the Ironman workout, don't stop there. Continue on and go back to the pec-deck machine, and do three sets of that exercise. This will bring you up to four chest exercises or twelve total sets—the required amount for the Ironman workout. If you are doing the Superman workout, don't stop there. Continue on and go back to the seated machine press, and do another three sets of that exercise. This will bring you up to five chest exercises or fifteen total sets—the required amount for the Superman workout.

Notice that you alternate exercises. Rather than do all of your seated machine press work, and then all of your pec-deck work, you switch back and forth, in order to give the body a brief change of pace. The system is simple, and can be used anytime you have a situation where there are only two available exercises for a given body part, and you want to do three or more exercises for that body part.

But what do you do if the machine is even more limited, and offers only one exercise for a body part? For example, in the above case, suppose there is only a seated machine press, but no pec-deck device. The answer is obvious. Use that one machine for all sets of your exercises. But treat each three sets as a separate exercise. In other words, pyramid your weights for the first three sets. Then go back to the lighter weight and pyramid your weights for the next three sets, and so on, until you have completed the required number of sets for your workout (nine sets for the regular workout, twelve sets for the Ironman workout, and fifteen sets for the Superman workout).

Sound boring? Of course it is. For this reason, if you are on the Ironman or Superman workout, no harm will be done if you switch to the regular workout for a few days, or even for a few weeks. You might find that doing more than nine sets of the same exercise for a given body part is just too much to tolerate.

Non-Total-Body Machines

What should you do in the case where the machine has no device for exercising a certain body part? For some body parts, you will have no problem, since no machines or free weights are needed. For example, you don't need any equipment to exercise your abdominals. All you have to do is follow the abdominal workout outlined in Chapter 6. But what about the other body parts? Let's look at each one of them separately.

All machines have chest-pressing devices, so you won't have to worry about that. As far as biceps go, all machines have lat-pulldown devices, and as you know, you can perform your machine biceps pulldown using the lat-pulldown device (see pp. 160–161). You can also use the lat-pulldown device to do the triceps pushdown, even if the only bar available is the lat-pulldown bar. You can improvise by gripping the bar with your hands six to eight inches apart, and performing the exercise exactly as described on p. 164. The only difference will be, you will be using the cumbersome lat-pulldown bar instead of a short straight or curved triceps bar.

As far as your back goes, you can of course do lat pulldowns, both wide and narrow grip (see pp. 176–177), and in fact, you can do lat pulldowns to the back with a wide grip for a third variation. (Simply pull the bar down behind your neck until it touches your rear shoulders.) For all other aspects of the exercises, follow the instructions for the lat pulldown to the front.

Most machines have one shoulder device. But if there is no such device, follow the in-the-room (see p. 201) workout for shoulders. Most hotel gyms have a seated leg press, so, if you are doing the optional leg workout, you can substitute your leg work for leg presses. Sit at the seat of the leg press machine, and do as many sets as necessary until you have completed the required number of sets for the routine you are performing (nine for the regular workout, twelve for the Ironman workout, and fifteen for the Superman workout). Remember to treat each three sets as a separate exercise, by pyramiding for the next three sets and then returning to a lighter weight and pyramiding for the next three sets and so on.

Calves can also be exercised on the seated leg press machine. Simply place the soles of your feet on the edge of the pressing device, and let the heels of your feet descend downward. Then press the weights by pushing with the soles of your feet, and when you cannot go any further, return to start position, and so on. You will be able to take all three positions—toes straight ahead, toes pointed outward, and toes pointed inward.

If the hotel gym machine does not have a leg press station, follow the in-the-room workout for these body parts (see p. 201).

Limited Free Weights and No Machines

If the hotel gym has a generous supply of free weights, or even if, by luck, the gym has three sets of dumbbells, and they are just the right weights for you, obviously, you have no problem. You can perform the workout found in Chapter 6. But what if that's not the case?

For example, what if the gym has only a few light sets of dumbbells—much lighter than the dumbbells you are used to using? Use the heaviest set of dumbbells for all three sets, and do ten repetitions for each set. Flex your muscles extra hard to make up for the lighter weights.

If the gym has only heavy dumbbells (usually not the case, since if dumbbells are provided, there are usually light ones for the female guests, but it can happen), use the heavy dumbbells if you can get a minimum of a comfortable four repetitions per set, and do three sets of four repetitions with that weight. If you can get more than four repetitions, pyramid the weights based upon the highest amount of repetitions you can get.

For example, if you can get six repetitions, do six repetitions for your first set, five repetitions for your second set, and four repetitions for your third set. If you can get eight repetitions, do eight repetitions for your first set, seven repetitions for your second set, and six repetitions for your last set, and so on.

Limited Free Weights and Non-Total-Body Machine

What if you find yourself in a situation where there are a few free weights around, but not the ideal weights, and also an incomplete machine. Simple. Create your own program by combining the methods discussed above. You now have enough knowlege to survive, even in the worst possible hotel gym situations. You'll be surprised at how quickly you become inventive.

When No Hotel Gym Is Available—In-the-Room Workout

Your best bet is to get a copy of *The 12-Minute Total-Body Workout* and carry it with you, just in case there is no hotel gym available. The book was written specifically for this purpose of working out quickly, and without equipment. It covers all body parts, so you can use it for only those body parts that are left out of the gym workout, or you can use if for an entire workout. If you use that book, you will make three changes from the book:

1. Double the daily workout by doing two workout days at a time. In other words, your in-the-room workout will take twenty-four minutes, rather than twelve minutes. Instead of doing just the Monday workout on Monday, you would do the Monday and Tuesday workout on Monday. Then you take one day off from working out, and the next time you work out, you would do the Wednesday and Thursday workout. Again, you would take one day off from working out, and the third time you work out, you would do the Friday and Saturday workout. Then you would repeat the pattern, so that you would work out three days a week.

   If you wish to do a shorter workout, and work out every day, simply follow the exact workout in the book. It will take you twelve minutes a day. This method is just as effective as the above method. You can make your decision based upon your available morning time. Which is more convenient for you— a twelve-minute daily workout when you are on the road, or a twenty-four-minute, three-day-a-week workout?

2. The book asks the exerciser to use three-pound dumbbells, but you don't have to use them. Since the writing of that book, I have discovered that weights are not necessary. All that is needed are the exercise movements and isometric pressure and dynamic tension (clearly described in that book). If you feel better using the three-pound weights, however, deflatable water weights that are ideal for travel are now available, and can be ordered by calling CAEF Inc. at 1-800-251-6040.

3. Leave out the hip/buttocks exercises. They are specifically designed for women.

What if you don't have a copy of *The 12-Minute Total-Body Workout*? Then do your regular Top Shape Workout in your room, without weights. What? Am I kidding? Of course not. It works. But you'll have to compensate for the lack of weights by using the isometric pressure and dynamic tension method described in *The 12-Minute Total-Body Workout*. In case you don't want to read that book, let me explain the method here.

An isometric movement involves the tensing of one set of muscles in opposition to another set of muscles. In a sense, it is simply a continual "flex," or to put it another way, it is continual peak contraction. To understand the way isometric pressure is used, lower your right arm down at your side until it is fully extended downward. Make a fist. Now, flex your biceps muscle by clenching your fist as hard as possible. Now, continuing to flex that muscle as hard as possible, raise your arm by bending at the elbow, and as you raise it, continue to flex your biceps muscle as hard as possible. This is isometric pressure—continual flexing, or continual peak contraction.

Right now you may be thinking, "Didn't I just read in the Top Shape Workout exercise instructions that I should do the same thing?" How is this different? It is very different, because when you are trying to flex a muscle while lifting a weight, you can only flex so much. Your muscle needs some of its strength to handle the heaviness of the weight. When you are trying to flex a muscle with no weight, you can really get a maximum flex, and in fact, if you are working without weights, the entire efficacy of your workout depends upon how hard you flex, or how much isometric pressure you use.

Dynamic tension, the other principle involved in this system, follows the muscle through the stretching phase of the movement. Let's continue with the biceps curl example. Now that your arm is fully bent, and your biceps muscle completely flexed, begin to uncurl your arm by slowly extending it downward to your side. But instead of allowing the muscle to relax as you go, keep the pressure on the muscle.

How do you do this? You can't flex a muscle on the stretching movement, can you? No. But you can create tension. Here's how. Make believe that someone is trying to hold your arm up in the bent position, and that you are trying with all of your might to uncurl your arm. You will quickly see how much work, or "tension," you put on the muscle. In other words, rather than allow the muscle fibers to lie stagnant during what would otherwise be a relaxing phase of the movement, the extension or stretching phase, you cause your muscle fibers to work—to be "dynamic." You create "dynamic tension."

Continuing the example, you would keep up the dynamic tension on your biceps muscle as you uncurl your arm, until your arm is fully extended at your side and back to start position. At this point your biceps muscle will be fully stretched. You would continue to perform each repetition in this manner, using isometric pressure and dynamic tension, until you have completed your set. A more complete discussion of this method is found in *The 12-Minute Total-Body Workout*, but for now, suffice it to say that if you use the method, not only will you keep your muscles in shape until you return to your regular workout, but you will achieve additional definition and hardness.

Since you will not be using weights, and obviously will not be using the pyramid system, you will do all three sets of your in-the-room Top Shape Workout with ten repetitions.

Use the In-the-Room Method for Select Body Parts

If you are not using the in-the-room method for your entire workout, but just for certain body parts that you had to skip in the hotel gym because no appropriate exercise apparatus was available, simply perform your Top Shape Workout for that body part only, using the method described above.

DOING AEROBIC EXERCISE ON THE ROAD

Before we even discuss aerobic options, I want to make it crystal clear that you must not replace your Top Shape Workout with an aerobic workout. Your Top Shape Workout comes first. Once you have done that, then you can (and in fact you should) do aerobics. (See p. 66 for a discussion of the reasons for this mandate.)

If there is a hotel gym, chances are, shamefully, even if it has no weights or machines, it will have a few pieces of aerobic equipment. You can do a twenty-to-thirty-minute workout on any piece of aerobic equipment—an exercise bike (any brand), a stair-stepper, a treadmill, a rowing machine, a NordicTrack machine, and so on. You don't have to be fussy. As long as it is an aerobic piece of equipment, you can use it.

If there is no aerobic equipment available, and you don't mind leaving the hotel, you can go outside and run in one direction for ten to fifteen minutes, and then turn around and go back. You will have run for a total of twenty minutes. If you don't like to run, you can walk at a fast pace for double the time (it takes twice the time in walking to equate running in terms of fat burning).

I've saved the best aerobic option for last. You can get your aerobics out of the way in the privacy of your own room. If you carry a simple, inexpensive jump rope (it's very light in weight and it doesn't take up much space), you can jump rope for twenty to thirty minutes in the morning while watching the news on television, or while listening to the radio and thinking about the day ahead of you. (See p. 240 for information on purchasing a jump rope.)

YOU MAY HAVE TO BREAK INTO A NEW AEROBIC ACTIVITY SLOWLY

Even if you are already doing one aerobic activity, such as running on a treadmill, for example, and can perform that activity for thirty minutes without a problem, you will probably find that you cannot simply substitute that activity for another, and do it the first day for the same length of time.

For example, I regularly run for thirty-minute sessions. But the first time I tried to jump rope for thirty minutes, I had the devil of a time. The most I could do for the first session was five minutes. Then I increased my time by five minutes a day, until in six days I was jumping for thirty minutes straight. On the other hand, I was able to do ten minutes the first time I tried the stair-stepper, and fifteen minutes for my first exercise bike session.

Taking the above into consideration, if you want to be sure to get a full aerobic session in, why not break in ahead of time with a jump rope. This way you have a guarantee that no matter what, you can do your aerobics in your room.

KEEPING UP YOUR LOW-FAT EATING PLAN ON THE ROAD

There's no reason whatsoever to fear that you will be forced to give up low-fat eating (see Chapter 9) when you are away from home. No matter where you are in the world, there is a way to eat right when on the road. Your first consideration will be dining out in restaurants and dealing with hotel room service. Your next concern will be eating on the run, when no restaurant is available. You'll also have to deal with picking and choosing from buffet tables in meeting situations, and finally, you'll have to deal with airline food.

Dining Out in Restaurants

There is always something that you can order. Let's take each meal at a time.

Breakfast. All hotels serve poached or hard-boiled eggs. You can order one poached egg on whole wheat toast without the butter, or you can order three or four hard-boiled eggs, and eat only one yolk, but all the whites, and have a slice or two of whole wheat toast without the butter.

Another breakfast idea is a bagel or English muffin (regular white flour is fine for the road). You can eat it dry, ask for no-fat cream cheese (unlikely that they will have it, but you can try), or put a tablespoon of jam or jelly on it. You may also treat yourself to the slightly higher in fat corn muffin or bran muffin on occasion.

Finally, you are always safe with any bran or cornflakes-type of cold cereal, or a hot cereal such as oatmeal, farina, or Wheatena, as long as they assure you that it is cooked without butter.

Lunch. All hotels have lettuce and tomatoes, so you can order a large tossed salad, and ask for plain or wine vinegar (no oil included) on the side. If you don't have a sodium problem, you can order a bowl of vegetable or chicken with rice or noodle soup. When you get it, spoon out any visible oil from the top.

Next, you can order a cold breast of chicken or turkey, and you can remove the skin, or, you can order a chicken or turkey breast sandwich with mustard, or have it dry, with lettuce and tomatoes.

There is usually a cottage cheese selection offered in the diet section of the menu, but beware. Ask if the cottage cheese is low-fat. If it isn't, there will be four grams of fat per ounce—sixteen grams of fat per four-ounce serving. If you're going to have that much fat, you might as well enjoy a chicken salad sandwich—for about the same amount of fat in the mayonnaise.

You can have fresh fruits or fruits in their own juices for dessert.

Dinner. As an appetizer, you can have a shrimp cocktail (low in fat but a little high in cholesterol) or a tossed salad.

Almost any restaurant will serve you a plain baked potato or steamed rice, without any butter, or plain pasta with no sauce on it. If the restaurant assures you that the pasta has a marinara sauce that is not high in fat, you can try it.

For a main dish, you can order flounder, sole, or any of the low-fat fish mentioned on pp. 215–216. But ask for them broiled, baked, or steamed without any butter or oil. You may also have white-meat chicken or turkey served the same way.

You can order any vegetable, but ask them to cook it without butter. If they can't do that, toss the vegetables around in a few paper napkins to remove the excess butter. For dessert, you can ask for low-fat frozen yogurt, or order assorted fresh berries.

Ordering Room Service

If you are eating one of your meals in, if it is still the normal mealtime, you can usually order from the same menu offered by the restaurant. If this is the case, follow the above guidelines.

If you're ordering from the limited room service menu, and are looking for a snack, you can order some fruit or a bowl of pretzels (not potato chips or chips of any kind). If you're feeling extra hungry, you can also order "odd things," like two baked potatoes and a serving or two of green beans and carrots, or some such thing.

There will be all sorts of salads listed. Ask about the particular contents of the salad, and perhaps you can bargain with the cook to double up one item for an item you want left out. For example, most chef's salads contain lettuce and tomatoes, eggs, white-meat chicken, ham, and roast beef. You may be able to convince the cook to give you triple the chicken and leave out the roast beef and ham. If you can't, then you can always remove the roast beef and ham once you get the salad.

KEEP IT SIMPLE

If you want to be on the safe side, stick to the simple foods. Avoid foods with strange names. You can be sure they are probably mixed with a generous supply of fat or oil. In any case, if you do want to take a chance, you will have to quiz the waiter at length as to the restaurant's willingness to cook the food for you without butter or oil.

Don't order anything stir-fried. It has plenty of oil and the fat grams will put you over your limit. Avoid "salads" of tuna, chicken, or shrimp or pasta. They are always replete with high-fat mayonnaise or oil.

Eating on the Run

If you know that you are going to have a busy day, and will not have time to stop for a meal, think ahead. Stop off in a deli or grocery store and get a white-meat turkey or chicken sandwich on whole wheat bread with mustard, and a couple of pieces of fruit. You can also buy some raw vegetables such as carrots, cucumbers, or red peppers. Another idea is to buy a couple of bagels or a bag of pretzels. You can also pick up a few cans of tuna in water and eat it out of the can. Low or no-fat yogurt or cottage cheese is not out of the question. Although these items are perishable, they will remain fresh out of the refrigerator if the temperature is below sixty-five degrees outside, and you keep the yogurt or cottage cheese in your car. Of course you can stock up on water or no-calorie drinks.

If you're not traveling with a car, using the rules above, you can ask the hotel to make you up something for the road. Remember, it's worth the small investment in time. If you think ahead, you can be in control of what happens to you. It's your life we're talking about. It's important.

Picking and Choosing from Buffet Tables

Follow the same rules you would follow for restaurant dining. Choose the fresh fruits and salads. Go for the vegetables, the chicken, the fish. If everything is swimming in oil or butter, use the blotting system. If the food selection is really bad, you can always fill up on bread. It's a lot better than eating a lot of high-fat foods.

Ordering Special Meals When Traveling by Plane

Most airlines offer special meals. Your best bet is to order the low-fat meal. You can't go wrong by doing that. If they don't offer a low-fat meal, your next-best bet is to order a low-calorie meal, because chances are, if it is low in calories, it will be low in fat.

If you forget to order a special meal, or, as is the case all too often, the airline does not have your special meal even though you ordered it, don't despair. You can still eat the food that is served, only choose the lesser of two evils if there is a choice, and then pick and choose what you eat from the meal that is served.

For example, a typical breakfast choice is often french toast or cold cereal. The answer is obvious. Choose the cold cereal. Most airlines offer low-fat milk these days, but even if they don't you're still better off with the cold cereal than with the fatty french toast. You could use a small amount of full-fat milk, or eat the cereal dry. Breakfast is usually served with a piece of fruit, so you are in luck there.

If you run into the lunch or dinner menu, stick to the restaurant guidelines. Pick chicken over beef. Blot the butter-laden vegetables. Eat the salad without the dressing. Eat the dinner roll without the butter. You can survive quite well when you know what you're doing.

A FINAL WORD ABOUT THE ROAD

A lot of people hate to travel because they think that on-the-road eating means inevitable weight gain. In fact, the opposite can easily be true. On the road, you have no available refrigerator. This fact alone can cause a weight loss rather than a weight gain, especially if you do a lot of snacking at home.

If you want to make sure you lose weight on the road, refuse the key to the mini-bar. It is usually filled with tempting high-fat treats such as peanuts, chips of every kind, and cookies. Sometimes, if you're lucky, you will find a bag of pretzels in a mini-bar, but unless you have excellent self-control, don't chance it. It's better to keep it locked.

Also, refrain from ordering from room service for that late-night snack. Go to bed with an empty stomach for a change. You'll feel great in the morning.

If you follow these rules, you'd be surprised to find that you can actually lose weight on the road. I've spoken to many people who, using the guidelines in this chapter, have done just that. (I for one always lose weight when I travel.)

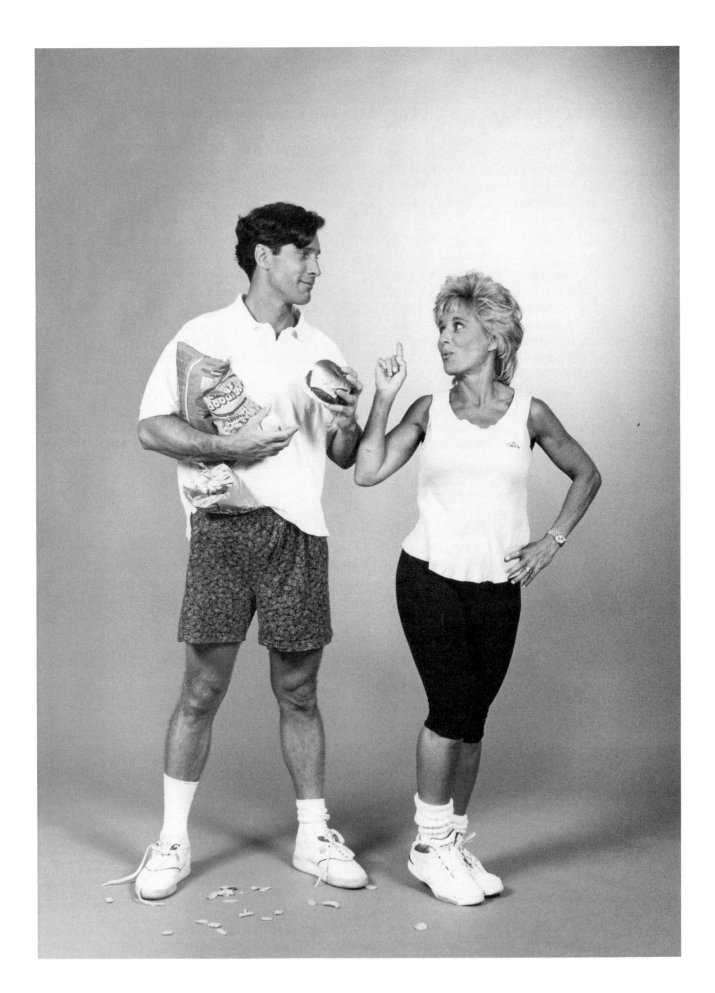

9

Top Shape Eating!

The best part of this diet is, it's not a diet," says one of the before-and-after men. "I used to fear food—try to eat only one meal a day. Now I eat five times a day, eat out, and I'm never hungry. I can eat like a human being. It's the easiest diet I've been on—not a punishment at all—and with the workout, I've been feeling so much energy."

You don't have to starve yourself in order to be in top shape. All you have to do is cut down on your fat intake and eat a well-balanced combination of foods. You get to eat plenty of pasta, baked potatoes, rice, bread, low-fat fish and poultry, fresh and frozen vegetables and fruits. Soon your body will crave these nutritious foods and, in fact, it will cry out in protest if you try to stuff it with fatty foods.

"After only two weeks of the diet," says one man on the program, "I tried to cheat a little and eat a couple of greasy meatballs cooked in fatty sauce and I was repulsed by it. I used to crave cheese—now I rarely think about it. Now I actually crave healthy foods. Every other diet I started for the past ten years, I'd go off it and that's it. But with this plan, if I go off it, I do my workout anyway, and then, before you know it, I go back on the diet because my body nags me to eat healthy again."

It's true. All of it. The diet is not a punishment—you get to eat plenty. Your body does become addicted to healthy foods, the workout itself pushes you to follow the diet—it tells you that you are "in training," and demands that you cooperate by giving it nutritious, muscle-building foods. And perhaps the best part of it all is, you don't have to count calories. All you have to do is to keep your fat grams down to between thirty and forty a day.

HOW WE LOSE AND GAIN WEIGHT

A calorie is a unit of chemical energy released to your body when you eat, and then digest food. We use this energy as fuel to breathe, walk, talk, exercise, and so on. When we consume just enough calories to sustain our body's daily needs, our weight remains stable, but when we consume more calories than we need to sustain our body's daily needs, we gain weight, or, to be more specific, our bodies begin to store the excess calories in the form of fat.

It takes a calorie deficit of 3,500 calories to use up one pound of this stored fat—a deficit that can be created by either exercising more, putting more muscle on the body (this raises the metabolism), consuming fewer calories (especially fat calories), or a combination of all three. The Top Shape Workout takes care of the first two elements. The low-fat eating plan contained in this chapter takes care of the third—for a winning fat-loss combination.

THE DIFFERENCE BETWEEN FAT CALORIES AND OTHER CALORIES

Fat calories cause your body to gain more weight, or to get fatter, than do other calories for two reasons:

1. They are compressed, In other words, you get more of them for your money—just what you don't need! For example, there are nine calories in one gram of fat—but there are only four calories in one gram of carbohydrate or protein.

2. When you consume fat, only 3 percent of that fat is used up in the digestion process, but when you consume protein or carbohydrate, about 20 percent of the calories are used up in the digestion process. In other words, for every hundred calories of fat you consume, ninety-seven of them are available for use or for fat storage, but for every hundred calories of pure protein or carbohydrate you consume, only eighty of those calories are available for use or fat storage. Simply put, it is better to eat a baked potato that is one hundred calories, but all carbohydrate and no fat, than it is to eat one third of a cup of ice cream that is one hundred calories but all fat! (Not to mention that the potato is high in density, and will satisfy your hunger, whereas you would have to eat two cups of ice cream to feel full. Food density will be discussed later in this chapter.)

WHY WE CANNOT TOTALLY ELIMINATE FAT FROM THE DIET

The human body needs a certain amount of fat in the diet in order to survive. The cell membranes and sex hormones are composed of a good deal of fat, and it is fat that cushions the internal organs. In addition, fat helps the body to absorb and make use of calcium and vitamins D, E, A, and K.

But don't worry. It's highly unlikely that you will have a fat deficiency in your diet. The average American consumes up to 50 percent of fat or well over one hundred grams of fat per day. You, on the other hand, will consume about 12 percent to 14 percent of your daily caloric intake in fat—from thirty to forty grams per day.

FAT IS FAT—WHETHER SATURATED OR POLYUNSATURATED—AND IN PLAIN ENGLISH, IT WILL MAKE YOU FAT IF YOU EAT IT!

Saturated and Unsaturated Fat

Saturated fats are considered unhealthy because they can raise your cholesterol level. These fats are found mainly in animal products such as meat, full-fat milk, cheese, and in butter, and in coconut oil. Except for coconut oil, they all become solid at room temperature.

Unsaturated fatty acids are considered to be less unhealthy because they do not raise your cholesterol level. They are liquid in form, and are derived from nuts, seeds, and vegetables. But these fats will make you just as fat as will saturated fats! In addition, research now shows that even these fats, if consumed in excess, cause a multiplicity of health problems.

FAT BANDITS!

You must avoid all fat in general, but here is a list of the most notorious "fat bandits:"

butter, margarine, oil, lard, or chicken fat
mayonnaise
peanut butter

ice cream, sour cream, cream cheese, whole milk
cheese of any kind
bacon, beef, lamb, and veal
all fried foods
all nuts and seeds
olives, avocados
chocolate, donuts
potato chips, corn chips, or any other kind of chips

By way of example, one tablespoon of butter, margarine, oil, or chicken fat contains an average of fourteen grams of fat—almost half your fat allowance for the day. Cheese averages ten grams of fat per slice—and most people eat at least four slices at a sitting—a grand total of forty grams of fat—your maximum fat allotment for the day. Six ounces of even the leanest hamburger will be about twenty grams of fat, and if you indulge in six ounces of sausage, you've more than doubled your fat allowance for the day—sixty-two grams of fat. And take a look at the fat contained in these quick-snack junk foods:

QUICK-SNACK JUNK FOODS	FAT GRAMS
4 ounces potato chips	45
4 ounces tortilla chips	30
4 ounces peanuts	35
10 chocolate sandwich cookies	34
1 donut	27
McDonald's apple pie	14
chocolate candy bar	15
croissant	11
large Dairy Queen ice cream dipped in chocolate	20
chocolate milkshake	10
Burger King regular onion rings	15
Burger King regular french fries	22
hot dog	15
4 ounces refried beans with sausage	32
Jack in the Box super taco	17
Burger King double cheeseburger	32
Burger King Whopper	36
Arby's super roast beef sandwich	28
Arby's turkey sandwich	24
Arthur Treacher's fish sandwich	19.2
McDonald's Egg McMuffin	14
Taco Bell beef burrito	20
Wendy's baked potato with cheese	24
Wendy's baked potato plain	2 (for contrast)

For a quick guideline as to the fat content in foods, get a copy of *The T-Factor Fat Gram Counter*. For a more comprehensive guide of the total food content of all foods, and for a very important reference book, get a copy of *The Nutrition Almanac*. These books are listed in the bibliography.

A GIFT: PIZZA IN AN EMERGENCY!

Pizza has often been grouped with junk snacks; however, it is not nearly as bad as those listed above. For example, one slice of plain pizza, especially if you blot off the excess oil, is only about five grams of fat. So in an emergency, if you count the fat grams into your daily allotment, and if you're honest with yourself and you don't order double cheese, but rather ask for more tomatoes, and if you do a good job of blotting off the excess oil, you can have a slice of pizza!

WHAT ABOUT CHOLESTEROL?

Cholesterol is not fat. It is a fatlike substance that can clog the arteries, and is found in fatty foods as well as nonfatty foods. For example, there is quite a bit of cholesterol in very low-fat seafood, and also a lot of cholesterol in beef, a very high-fat meat.

Like fat, cholesterol is not all bad. It is a component of cell membranes and nerve linings, and is found in the brain, liver, and blood. It also helps to form the sex and adrenal hormones, vitamin D, and bile.

The body naturally produces its own cholesterol, so you don't have to worry about getting enough cholesterol in your diet. You do, however, have to worry about getting too much of it in your diet. Here's why.

When there is too much LDL cholesterol in the blood (which has come to be labeled "bad" cholesterol), arteries can be clogged and you can suffer a heart attack. Here's how it works. If an overabundance of LDL is carried through the arterial walls, it eventually becomes deposited on the arterial walls as plaque, causing the arterial walls to become too narrow to allow blood to freely pass through them, causing undue pressure on the heart. Eventually, the pressure that is put upon the heart can cause all kinds of heart problems, up to and including a fatal heart attack.

HDL is called "good" cholesterol because it removes cholesterol from the bloodstream and helps transport LDL out of the cells, into the bile, and into the intestines where it is eventually excreted out of the body.

It's Not the Total Cholesterol but the Ratio That Counts

In order to find out if you are "in trouble," it's not enough to know only your total cholesterol count, because you would have no way of knowing how much good (HDL) cholesterol you have, as opposed to how much bad (LDL), troublemaking cholesterol you have. You must find out the ratio!

In order to find out your ratio of good (HDL) to bad (LDL) cholesterol, you must get a "fractionated" cholesterol test. This will give you what is called an "index." The lower your index, the lower your risk (an index of 4 or lower is considered low-risk). For example, if your total cholesterol level is 200, and your HDL is 50, your index is 4 (a safe, low index). If on the other hand, your total cholesterol level is 200, but your HDL level is only 25, you are at risk, because your index is high, an 8!

Your goal, then, is to raise your HDL and lower your LDL. You can raise HDL by doing this workout and/or other regular exercise, and you can lower the bad LDL by limiting your consumption of saturated fats, alcohol, refined sugars, caffeine, and, if you are a smoker, by quitting.

PROTEIN: EAT TWO TO THREE PORTIONS OF PROTEIN PER DAY

Protein is the main building and repairing material of muscles, bones, hair, fingernails, skin, ligaments, enzymes, blood, immune cells, and internal organs. In fact, muscles are composed mainly of protein.

Protein also plays a role in regulating the acid-alkaline balance of the blood and tissues, and in regulating the body's water balance. It is an essential element in the production of hormones that control metabolism, growth, and sexual development.

When protein is digested, it is broken down into smaller units called "amino acids." Fourteen of these twenty-two amino acids can be produced by the human body without the aid of an outside source, but the remaining eight must be obtained from special foods called "complete protein," or "essential amino acids." They are found in fish, poultry, beef, egg whites, yogurt, or legumes such as lentils, split peas, or beans (vegetarians must combine nonmeat protein with rice, corn, or milk to make up complete protein).

Daily Protein Intake

Unlike fat, protein cannot be stored, so we must feed our body a small amount of protein at a time—about thirty grams per sitting. A bare minimum of total daily protein consumption is about fifty-five grams. Since you will be building muscle with this program, you will be allowed to eat more than that (people who work with weights can consume up to one half gram daily per pound of body weight).

For example, if you weigh 160 pounds, and you work out with weights, you can consume a maximum of eighty grams of protein per day. On the other hand, you don't have to keep your protein that high. You can go as low as fifty-six grams per day (as recommended for men by the Pritikin Longevity Center), and no harm will be done. My only reason for suggesting slightly higher protein is, when you're building muscle, your body seems to like more protein. I can't prove this, except to say that all bodybuilders consume half their weight in protein because they say their muscles thrive on it (keep in mind that a bodybuilder may weigh 260 pounds, and that his protein intake would be 130 grams per day, whereas if you followed the half-gram protein per pound of body weight, and you weigh, say 160 pounds, your daily intake would be much lower—80 grams per day).

LOW-FAT PROTEIN IS THE KEY: EAT THIRTY TO FORTY GRAMS OF FAT PER DAY

For our purposes, one portion of protein is six to eight ounces of poultry or fish, six to eight ounces of yogurt, cottage cheese, or tofu, one half to two thirds cup of beans, or three to five egg whites. Note that the protein grams in these portions vary, allowing you to decide how much protein you want to consume in a given day.

You will get your protein from white-meat poultry, low-fat fish, cottage cheese, beans, tofu, and egg whites. Let's discuss poultry and fish first.

Poultry and Fish

There is about one gram of fat per ounce of white-meat poultry, and about five grams of protein. If you remove the skin from the poultry, and remember not to eat anything that is fried, white-meat poultry is an excellent source of protein. (Leaving the skin on poultry and eating it fried increases the fat grams per ounce to four grams—that's a 400 percent increase! If you're going to do that, why fool yourself into believing you are eating a low-fat diet? You might as well eat beef—which contains less fat per ounce—an average of only two and one half grams of fat per ounce.)

Most fish is a lot lower in fat than even low-fat poultry, so when it comes to a low-fat source of protein, fish is a real food bargain. For example, *four* ounces of the following fish are lower in fat or the same as *one* ounce of poultry, yet both poultry and fish yield about the same amount of protein per ounce—five grams.

4 OUNCES OF FISH	FAT GRAMS
Haddock	0.5
Red snapper	0.5
Cod	0.6
Abalone	0.6
Sea bass	1.0

And *four* ounces of the following fish are lower in fat or the same as *two* ounces of poultry:

4 OUNCES OF FISH	FAT GRAMS
Sole	1.6
Flounder	1.6
Squid	1.8
Tuna in water	2.0
Pike	2.0

Don't be fooled. Some fish is high in fat, and should be avoided while you are trying to lose weight. Later, once you reach your goal, you can incorporate them into your diet from time to time.

4 OUNCES OF FISH	FAT GRAMS
Salmon	7.4
Swordfish	8.0

Cottage Cheese, Yogurt, Egg Whites, and Tofu

There is only one gram of fat in four ounces of 1 percent low-fat cottage cheese, and no fat at all in no-fat cottage cheese, and two grams of protein. The same amount of full-fat cottage cheese, on the other hand, contains five grams of fat, but you only get the same two grams of protein for your money!

Low-fat yogurt contains about one and one half grams of fat for four ounces, and has about six grams of protein. Three egg whites have no fat at all, yet they contain ten grams of protein. Four ounces of tofu contain about four and one half ounces of fat, and contain eight ounces of protein. (Note that tofu is a borderline low-fat food source. If you choose it, be aware.)

WHAT ABOUT NO-FAT FOOD PRODUCTS?

It is always better to choose a no-fat food over low-fat food, but you must be careful not to abuse the food by overindulging—just because you know it has no fat. Even though you are not counting calories, but fat grams, if you make it a goal, you could probably gain weight on a low-fat diet. Let me explain.

A no-fat substitute for fat, Simplesse, is made of the proteins from egg whites in combination with no-fat milk products, and is now used in no-fat cottage cheese. If you ate ten eight-ounce containers of it a day, even though it has no fat, you would still consume about 1,400 calories (about seventy calories for a four-ounce serving). This alone would not make you gain weight, but if you did the same thing with no-fat desserts such as ice cream and cake, you can see where you would raise your calorie intake to the point where your body would have no choice but to store it as fat.

On the other hand, you can also see (as you must be thinking by now) how unlikely it would be that you would even dream of eating ten containers of cottage cheese, or 'ten cups of no-fat ice cream, or anything similar. So you can see here why the low-fat eating plan generally works—without counting calories.

CARBOHYDRATES

Carbohydrates are the main source of energy to your body and your brain. If you deprive your body of carbohydrates, not only do you feel weak, you literally cannot think straight.

Carbohydrates include a large category of foods: simple carbohydrates (sugars), which break down into two groups: refined and unrefined. Sugars in candy and cake are refined, and sugars in fruit are unrefined. Complex carbohydrates include vegetables, grains, and fiber.

Complex carbohydrates provide gradually released energy, while simple, unrefined carbohydrates (fruits) provide immediate energy.

IS SUGAR (REFINED SIMPLE CARBOHYDRATES) AS BAD AS FAT?

Sugar will not make you as fat as fat, but you must limit your sugar intake anyway, because if you consume it in excess, too much glucose is released into your bloodstream, and this will cause your body to produce high levels of insulin, which hinders hormone-sensitive lipase, the enzyme that is responsible for pulling fat from the fat cells. In short, too much sugar can cause your body to resist giving up its fat cells.

Another problem with sugar is, it can stimulate your appetite. If you consume it in excess, the resulting overproduction of insulin causes blood sugar to go directly to the liver, creating a blood sugar deficit in the circulatory system. End result? A sense of weakness that is usually interpreted by the body as hunger.

FRUIT AND FRUIT JUICE: UNREFINED SIMPLE SUGARS— MUCH BETTER THAN REFINED SIMPLE SUGARS, BUT BE AWARE

Even though fruits are not refined sugars, they are still simple sugars and are converted into glucose (potential energy) quickly—more quickly than complex carbohydrates. Like refined sugars, fruits give a quick energy boost and then a drop in energy if you eat them on an empty stomach, but they are better than simple refined sugars that do the same thing, because fruits contain fiber and vitamins, and because the sugar in a fruit is not as concentrated as the sugar in, say, a candy bar, and so will not give you quite the same energy boost and dramatic letdown.

Fruit juice is another matter. It is a more concentrated dose of simple sugar than fruit—mainly because one usually consumes more than the equivalent of one piece of fruit when one drinks juice, and also because there is no food bulk to absorb the sudden dose of simple sugar. In addition, fruit juice as compared to fruit is a poor food bargain, because one cannot feel full by drinking a glass of juice, whereas one can feel quite full after eating, say, two apples.

EAT THREE TO FOUR FRUITS PER DAY

You will be allowed to have three to four fruits a day. Each of the following constitutes one serving of fruit:

1 large apple	¼ large pineapple	1 large nectarine
4 apricots	½ large plantain	1 large orange
1 small banana	1½ cups strawberries	1 large peach
1 cup berries (any kind)	1½ cups watermelon	3 persimmons
½ cantaloupe	20 grapes	2 plums
15 large cherries	¼ honeydew melon	3 fresh prunes
½ grapefruit	1 large kiwifruit	2 tangerines
1 cup papaya	3 kumquats	
1 medium pear	1 small mango	

If you discover other fruits not listed here, by all means indulge in them. If you are in doubt about their nutrutional content, look it up in *The Nutrition Almanac* (see bibliography).

FOODS IN LOW-CALORIC DENSITY: A REAL FOOD BARGAIN

All things considered, if you are tying to lose weight, it's better to eat a food that will fill your stomach than one that is light and airy, and will leave your stomach feeling slightly empty. For example, it is better to eat a bowl of oatmeal that is about eighty calories than it is to eat a bowl of cold cereal that has the same number of calories—without the milk.

Carrying this idea further, it is better to eat three cups of broccoli and cauliflower (about eighty calories) than it is to eat two slices of whole wheat bread—(also eighty calories) if your goal is to feel full and to prevent yourself from continually going back to pick.

Caloric density, the number of calories per weight of that particular food, is an important consideration when trying to lose weight. The human stomach can hold a maximum of two to three pounds of food at a time, so if you want to feel full, fill your stomach with low-calorie, high-density foods. Then your stomach will be too full to hold any more food and you will stop eating.

The following is a list of high-density foods that are the best calorie bargain for filling you up:

Vegetables of every kind   (potatoes, sweet potatoes, and yams are
                                    especially filling)

Whole grain pastas
Whole grain and brown rice
Oatmeal and other hot cereals

The caloric-density principle holds true for simple sugars too. You will feel more full if you eat half a cantaloupe than you will if you eat two tablespoons of jelly, and the cantaloupe will have half the calories of the jelly; and in the bargain, you will have gotten plenty of fiber and vitamins.

EAT AT LEAST TWO AND ONE HALF CUPS
OF UNLIMITED COMPLEX CARBOHYDRATES PER DAY,
AND EAT THEM ANYTIME YOU ARE HUNGRY

Medical experts agree that one of the best ways to remain healthy is to be sure to eat at least five servings (one half cup is a serving) of vegetables a day. For our purposes, this is wonderful news, because most vegetables fall into the unlimited complex carbohydrate category—and I want you to eat them anytime you are hungry—in addition to eating them at your meals. Here is a list:

Artichoke	Kale
Asparagus	Leeks
Beans—green or yellow	Lettuce
Broccoli	Mushrooms
Brussels sprouts	Okra
Cabbage	Onions
Carrots	Peppers—red or green
Celery	Radishes
Chickory	Rhubarb
Chinese cabbage	Rutabagas
Collard greens	Shallots
Cucumber	Spinach
Eggplant	Sprouts
Endive	Squash—zucchini or summer
Escarole	Tomatoes

EAT FOUR TO SIX PORTIONS OF LIMITED COMPLEX CARBOHYDRATES PER DAY

Some complex carbohydrates must be limited because of their relatively higher calorie content. Each of the following complex carbohydrates constitutes one serving:

1 cup corn or 1 large corn on the cob
½ to ⅔ cup beans or lentils of any kind
1 cup peas of any kind
1 cup winter squash
1 large potato, sweet potato, or yam
½ bagel (the condensed kind; the light, airy ones count as a whole bagel
    for one serving)
2 slices bread
2 ounces pretzels
1 English muffin
8 low-fat crackers
1 ounce dry or hot cereals (measured uncooked)
4 ounces pasta (measured dry)
¾ cup rice
4 rice cakes

It is best to eat whole grain, wheat, buckwheat, rye, cornmeal, or sourdough versions of the above, but you may from time to time indulge in the white bread varieties.

FIBER

Complex carbohydrates contain fiber. There are two types of fiber: soluble fiber (found in oat bran, psyllium, fresh fruits and vegetables, and legumes), which can be digested by the body, and insoluble fiber (found in whole wheat, whole grains, celery, corn, corn bran, green beans, green leafy vegetables, potato skins, and brown rice), which cannot be digested by the body.

Soluble fiber helps to lower blood sugar by slowing down the body's absorbtion of carbohydrates and preventing an insulin rush. It also helps to lower cholesterol levels by connecting with bile acids and escorting the cholesterol out of the body.

Insoluble fiber, so called because it cannot be digested by the human body, and is eliminated in the stool, supplies the stool with volume, which helps prevent constipation and possible colon and rectal cancer. In addition, insoluble fiber acts

221

as a fat vacuum. It actually helps to move fat out of the body. Because insoluble fiber cannot be digested by the human body, it passes through the digestive tract, and along the way it pulls some fat with it, until both are eliminated in the stool.

The FDA recommends a minimum of thirty grams of fiber per day. High fiber foods are:

GRAINS	GRAMS FIBER
1 ounce bran flakes-type cereal	9
1 slice whole wheat bread	2
1 slice cracked wheat bread	2
1 slice rye bread	1
(In contrast, a slice of white bread has only half a gram of fiber.)	

FRESH FRUITS	GRAMS FIBER
1 orange	5
1 pear	5
1 banana	4
1 cup strawberries	5
1 apple	3.5

FRESH VEGETABLES (1 cup each)	GRAMS FIBER
Spinach	11
Peas	8
Corn	8
Broccoli	8
Carrots	5
Eggplant	5
Cabbage	4
Green beans	5
Tomato	4
Baked potato	6

BEANS AND LEGUMES (1 cup each)	GRAMS FIBER
Baked beans	21
Split peas	21
Lentils	18

VITAMINS AND MINERALS

It is always better to get your vitamins and minerals from food sources than from food supplements. In addition, taking too many vitamin and mineral supplements can cause an imbalance in the digestive system, and prevent the body from absorbing the vitamins and minerals in the foods you eat. Eat right. Then, if your doctor recommends vitamin and mineral supplements, by all means use them—but don't go overboard.

SODIUM

Sodium is an essential mineral. Together with potassium it helps to regulate body fluids and maintain the acid-alkali balances of the blood. Sodium is also responsible for muscle contraction; therefore, a lack of it in the diet can cause severe cramping and even muscle shrinkage.

People who are dieting usually keep their sodium level low for two reasons: First, if you have high blood pressure (and many overweight people do), it can cause problems. Second, it causes water retention (sodium holds about fifty times its own weight in water), and if you're dieting, the last thing you need is to feel heavy from water retention (in fact, high sodium in your diet can cause you to hold up to ten pounds of excessive water).

However, all of the above considered, sodium cannot make you fat. In fact, if you are on a diet, and your doctor has not restricted your sodium intake, you can from time to time indulge in high-sodium foods with no compunction. So what! You hold a little extra water for a few days. It isn't permanent. And perhaps that bag of salty pretzels or that can of full-sodium soup helped you to resist eating a donut! (True, you can get pretzels and soup that are low in sodium, but some people feel they just don't taste as good, and are therefore not a full treat.)

How much sodium should you consume in your diet? The FDA recommends a maximum daily consumption of 3,300 milligrams, but other health authorities suggest a much lower maximum of 1,600 milligrams daily. What should you do? If you keep your daily sodium intake at about 1,500 to 2,500 milligrams you will probably not retain excessive water.

This allows you more than enough sodium to enjoy a normal diet. For example, six ounces of chicken has about 130 milligrams of sodium, while six ounces of most fish have about 600 milligrams of sodium. A half cantaloupe has 25 milligrams, a lettuce and tomato salad 8 milligrams, and a baked potato 6 milligrams.

You don't have to count sodium milligrams unless you have a problem with blood pressure, and your doctor has advised you to keep your sodium low. If you want to keep your sodium low, for our purposes, it will be enough to simply avoid certain foods. For example, stay away from canned foods. They contain about 1,000 milligrams for eight ounces. Also watch out for diet dinners. They often have about 1,000 milligrams of sodium per serving. Anything smoked or pickled is also high in sodium, as is most Chinese food, unless you order it without the MSG. Also watch out for condiments such as mustard, ketchup, steak sauce, and Worcestershire sauce (500 to 1,000 milligrams per tablespoon).

Finally, give up the salt shaker habit. Each shake contains about 300 miligrams of sodium, and one commercial packet of salt contains 500 milligrams!

WATER

One of the best ways to flush out excessive sodium from your system is to drink lots of water. That's right. Ironically, water does not cause water retention—it prevents it.

You should drink six to eight eight-ounce glasses of water per day, because you must replace the three quarts of water your body loses daily through perspiration and excretion. You will get the rest of the water through fruits and vegetables, which are comprised of about 85 percent water, and by drinking other beverages such as soup, coffee, tea, soda, fruit juices.

More than half the weight of the human body is water. We could live for a month or longer without food, but we would die in a few days without water. It is the basis of all body fluids, including digestive juices, blood, urine, lymph, and perspiration. It is the primary carrier of nutrients throughout the body, and is involved in nearly every body function, including absorbtion, digestion, excretion, circulation, lubrication, and regulation of body temperature.

If you increase your water intake, you will immediately notice an improvement in your complexion. Your skin will appear healthier and more ruddy. In addition, water helps to curb your appetite. If you drink a glass of water before your meal, you will find that you eat less.

In addition, believe it or not, many times when we think we are hungry, we are really thirsty, and we mistake this feeling for the need for food. Since food contains water, and since we choose to give it food instead of water, our bodies make do. So the next time you think you are hungry, try drinking some water first. Then, in ten minutes, if you are still hungry, you can eat. But you may find that you are no longer hungry!

CAFFEINE

Unless your doctor has told you to avoid caffeine, you can have two to three cups of coffee a day. Caffeine's reputation varies from one year to the next, depending upon the latest study. In some people, it can causes heart irregularities, fibrocystic breast tissue, stress, decreased blood flow to the brain, nausea, insomnia, fast pulse, increased need to urinate, or raised cholesterol levels. If you don't have any of the above problems, and your doctor says it's okay, you may find that a moderate amount of caffeine daily will give you an energy boost just when you need it the most.

ALCOHOL

Alcohol, in moderation, if you can handle moderation, can be fine for you. In fact, researchers at Harvard's School of Public Health did a study of men aged forty to seventy-five over a two-year period, and discovered that those men who drank light to moderate amounts of alcohol (not more than one or two drinks a day) had a 25 percent to 40 percent lower chance of developing heart disease.

In my opinion, a glass or two of wine every day is too much. Drinking, in general, relaxes you to the point where your metabolism slows down. It's better to save your one or two drinks for the weekends. If you do drink, stick to the lower calorie beverages such as white or red wine, champagne, or hard liquor with plain soda or fruit juice.

THE FAT-LOSS EATING PLAN: WHAT YOU WILL EAT EVERY DAY

1. Consume no more than thirty to forty grams of fat per day. It is of course better to stay at the lower end of the scale. You will use up most of your fat allowance in your protein requirement.

2. Consume a minimum of fifty-five grams of protein per day, and up to one half your body weight in protein grams. Remember: there are approximately five or six grams of protein for every ounce of poultry or fish. Eat only white-meat poultry with the skin removed, and eat all fish or meat boiled, broiled, baked, steamed, or poached. Do not eat anything fried!

3. Eat four to six portions of limited complex carbohydrates per day.

4. Eat at least two and one half cups of unlimited complex carbohydrates per day—and more if you choose to do so.

5. If you are feeling extra hungry, choose complex carbohydrates that are high in density and low in calorie—such as oatmeal, pasta, vegetables.

6. Drink six to eight eight-ounce glasses of water per day. When you are hungry, drink a glass of water first. It will help to curb your appetite.

7. Never go more than five hours during the day without eating (it's better to eat every three to four hours). Cut the size of your meals, but eat more often.

SAMPLE DAILY MEAL PLANS FOR WEIGHT LOSS

Here are some sample meal plans. For additional suggestions, and interesting recipes, see bibliography under "Nutrition, Diet, Spas, and Cookbooks."

Note: Beverages are not listed. You may choose from any no-calorie beverage, such as seltzer, water, coffee, tea, no-calorie sodas.

SAMPLE DAILY MEAL PLAN NO. 1

Breakfast

1 toasted bagel and 1 tablespoon no-fat cream cheese
1 orange

Snack

1 banana
2 ounces pretzels

Lunch

6 to 8 ounces roasted chicken breast
1 cup green beans
tossed green salad
one dinner roll

Snack

1 cup blueberries

Dinner

6 to 8 ounces sole
1 cup broccoli and cauliflower
1 cup carrots
1 corn on the cob
tossed green salad

Snack

2 cucumbers and sliced red peppers
1 pear
bowl of oatmeal

SAMPLE DAILY MEAL PLAN NO. 2

Breakfast

Bowl of whole-grain cold cereal with skim milk
1 large peach

Snack

1 cup no or low-fat yogurt
1 cup grapes

Lunch

bowl low-fat vegetable soup
turkey breast sandwich on whole wheat bread with mustard
tossed green salad
mixed fruit salad in its own juice

Snack

2 sliced cucumbers
1 apple

Dinner

6 to 8 ounces sea bass
4 ounces pasta (dry) and 4 ounces low-fat tomato sauce
1 cup peas and carrots
1 cup spinach

Snack

8 wheat crackers
1 cup lentil soup
tossed green salad

SAMPLE DAILY MEAL PLAN NO. 3

Breakfast

1 egg yolk and 3 egg whites
½ cantaloupe
2 slices rye bread

Snack

1 cup low- or no-fat yogurt
1 cup strawberries

Lunch

4 to 6 ounces tuna in water on 2 slices of cracked wheat bread
sliced tomato
1 cup green beans
½ grapefruit

Snack

1 cup raspberries
2 slices of sourdough bread, toasted, with no-fat mayonnaise
    and lettuce and tomatoes (sandwich)

Dinner

6 to 8 ounces flounder
1 cup broccoli and cauliflower mix
1 cup Brussels sprouts
1 large baked potato and no-fat sour cream
large tossed green salad

Snack

1 cup Chinese vegetables
1 cup popcorn

I am well aware that you will be eating many of your meals out. For more information on this subject, read Chapter 8, "On the Road."

HOW MUCH WEIGHT CAN YOU EXPECT TO LOSE WITH THIS PLAN?

If you are about thirty to thirty-five pounds overweight, you can expect to lose about twenty to twenty-four pounds in twelve weeks—an average of about a pound and a half to two pounds a week—but you may lose a little more—due to the shift of water weight, or a little less—because while you are losing weight, your body is gaining muscle (a pound or two in three months' time).

Why so slow? It's not really slow when you come to think of it. After all, did you gain more than an average of two pounds a week when you were overeating and getting fat? There are fifty-two weeks in a year. Did you gain more than 104 pounds in a year? Of course not. Chances are you didn't gain more than a pound a week—fifty-two pounds a year, even though you were "working on it," by eating anything you wanted to eat, anytime you wanted to eat it. In fact, even working on it, you probably didn't gain more than thirty pounds in a year—a weekly weight gain of a little over a half a pound a week.

So don't be so impatient. Your body is cooperating with you by letting you lose the weight faster than you gained it, but as a survival system, your body cannot give up more than a pound or two of fat per week. (Some weeks the scale will show a larger drop than two pounds but that is usually water loss.) If you lose more than two pounds a week by starvation dieting, you will lose muscle in addition to fat (your body will begin to literally "eat" itself), and the moment you are off guard, your body will take over and force you to pig out and eat all of the high-fat foods you didn't eat before.

The end result will be not only fat gain, but change of body composition—you will now have a higher fat to muscle ratio because of lost muscle, and what's worse, you'll keep getting fatter because your metabolism will have slowed down! So when it comes to the body, don't try to beat the system. Your body is a system you can't beat. Stick to the nutritious, healthful way of losing weight. It's the only way to get it off and keep it off.

BUT WHAT IF YOU WANT TO GAIN WEIGHT?

Some men are too thin, and want to gain weight—not fat weight but muscle weight. In addition to weight-loss plans and recipes I have covered muscle-weight-gain plans extensively in my book *Supercut: Nutrition for the Ultimate Physique* (see bibliography). However, I'll give you a few simple guidelines here.

In order to gain weight, you'll have to eat high-quality protein that is a little higher in fat, and you'll have to increase your intake of complex and simple carbohydrates. You'll have to eat bigger meals, and even eat more often—a minimum of six times a day.

Here is a sample meal plan:

Meal 1

8 ounces milk
2 eggs
orange juice
2 slices toast and jelly

Meal 2

Corn muffin
1 cup dates

Meal 3

8 ounces roast chicken
2 cups wild rice
1 cup summer squash
milkshake

Meal 4

4 ounces tuna—in tuna salad sandwich
Tossed salad with one avocado in it

Meal 5

8 ounces lean hamburger
Mashed potatoes
1 cup vegetables
1 pear

Meal 6

1 cup fruity yogurt
½ cup nuts

Yes. You will be increasing your fat intake to over forty grams per day—but frankly, there is no other way to gain weight. But don't worry. Your fat intake will still be below 25 percent of your total fat consumption, the amount considered to by okay by the FDA.

If you are going to follow the above diet, it is crucial that you don't slack off on your weight-training program. In fact, it's a good idea to go on a split routine, and to work out four to six days a week, and, in addition, to use heavier weights (see p. 65 for this program).

HOW TO MAINTAIN YOUR WEIGHT: STICK TO THE GUIDELINES DURING THE WEEK, AND EAT WHATEVER YOU WANT ONE DAY A WEEK

Once you reach your weight goal, you can eat anything you want once a week—as long as you stick to the weight-loss guidelines in this chapter during the week.

How can this work? It's really not a mystery when you think of it. If you continued to follow the weight-loss plan forever, you would continue to lose weight forever. True, your weight loss would eventually slow down to as little as only an average of one eighth of a pound a week, but in time you would get thinner and thinner. The free eating day balances out the weight loss, and causes you to maintain your weight.

What should you eat on your free eating day? Anything you want—and you can do it all day long. I know what you're thinking. All week you'll gather your foods, and then have them at the ready. Then you'll get up at the crack of dawn and start eating—and you'll eat all day long—greasy hamburgers, thick shakes, donuts, ice cream, and so on. Well, try it. I did. And you know what, the next day I got so sick that by the next week I knew better than to try that again. I simply ate whatever I felt like eating—a lot of pizza, a bagel and plenty of cream cheese, and so on. The next day I felt fine.

The system works. In fact, some people can actually get away with pigging out two days a week—but I don't suggest that you experiment with this until you have been in top shape for a few years. By then, your body will be able to tell you how far you can go.

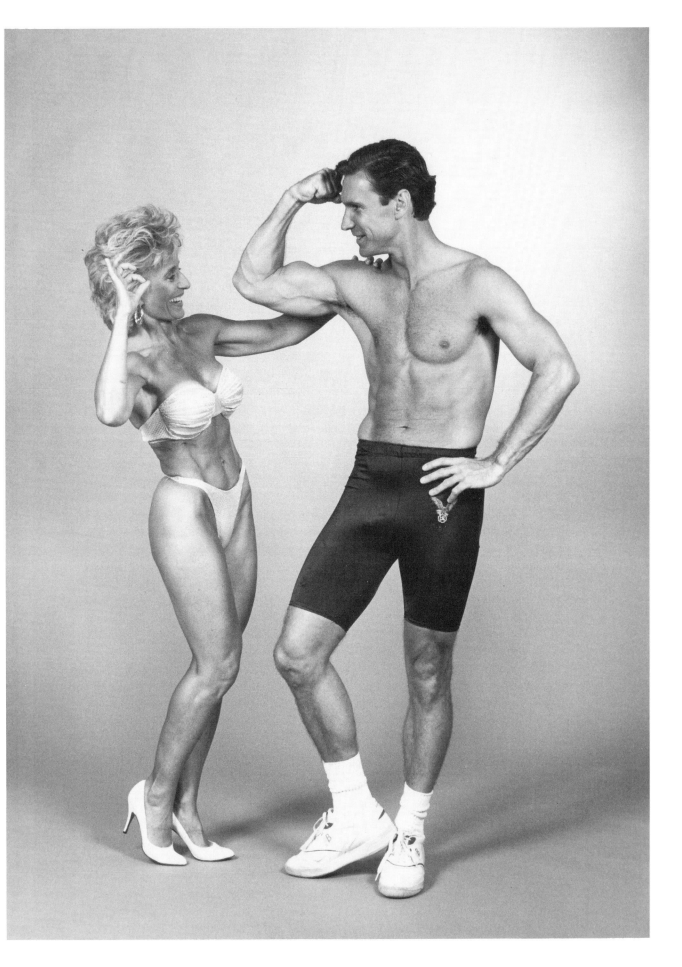

10

Maintaining It

Once you get into shape, you will never want to give up your workout—
or your new way of eating for that matter. Why? As you will soon find
out, the program is not a punishment, but rather a long-awaited relief for
your body—so instead of urging you to go off the program, your body will continually push you to stay with it.

After twelve weeks, when your body is composed of lean muscle instead of
unhealthy fat, and you have become accustomed to eating delicious, nutritious
low-fat foods, and working out, if you stopped working out, and/or started regularly
eating the wrong things, your body would remind you in no uncertain terms that
it is not happy. You would feel sluggish from not working out, and you would feel
nauseated from eating fatty foods.

GOING ON AUTOMATIC

After a while, the workout will become something you no longer have to think
about—like driving along a familiar route every day. For example, the first time
you drove to work, you had to pay attention, or you might have missed the exit,
turned down the wrong street, or passed the building. Now you don't have to think
about it. You just get in the car, and the car seems to drive itself. In fact, the ride
has become so automatic that you can practically do it in your sleep.

233

The same thing will happen with working out. It will become a part of your routine. Eventually, you will accept it as a necessary part of life—like brushing your teeth or taking a shower. It will no longer be something that is up for negotiation. Why? Because you will have seen that working out is as important as brushing your teeth or taking a shower. If you don't brush your teeth, decay sets in. If you don't take a shower, not only will you smell bad, but eventually you will have health problems (infections and even diseases). If you don't work out, eventually you will have health problems too.

In addition, just the way your mouth feels clean and fresh when you brush your teeth, and your body feels alive and renewed when you take a shower, your body will feel alert and powerful when you work out and eat right. So even if you tried to stop working out, your body would push you to start up again.

But how will you get to the point where you are on automatic? You will have to use discipline and sheer will. Use the tips found in Chapter 3 to motivate yourself to get started and to keep with the program. After that, while you are still in the beginning stages of the program, and you're tempted to quit, review that chapter, and think of the price versus the reward: three forty-minute sessions per week, and a low-fat eating plan that never asks you to be hungry versus a lifetime of fitness—not just externally (a handsome, muscular body) but internally (a healther heart and lungs, lower blood pressure, more energy, stronger bones, improved circulation and complexion). Is the price too high? Of course not. In fact, when you come to think of it, you'll probably decide that the Top Shape program is one of the best deals you've ever made, and you won't want to give it up for anything.

CAN YOU EVER TAKE A WEEK OFF?

What about time off? Do you have to work out week-in, week-out, month-in, month-out, year-in, year-out, without ever taking time off? Of course not. In fact, it's not a good idea to do that. The human body and mind need an occasional break. If this were not true, do you think that bosses would give their employees vacations?

You can take a week off every year—or even every six months if you so desire, but I don't advise you to take two weeks off at a time, because your body will feel as if such a long break is a punishment. As you know by now, you don't have to take time off if you are traveling for business, because you can always use the methods discussed in Chapter 8, "On the Road."

When you do take a week off from the Top Shape Workout, you don't have to stop exercising completely. After a day or two of vegetating, your body will propel you to at least move around a bit. After all, you've trained your body to thrive on exercise, so it isn't going to let you get away with complete stagnation. After you get your lying around and relaxing out of your system, go for a walk or a bike ride; play some tennis or go for a swim; do some water skiing or scuba diving. Do something—your body will appreciate it.

The best part of all of this is, when you do resume your workout, after about a week or two back on the program, your body will look better than it did had you not taken the time off at all. There seems to be a survival instinct in the body. When you take time off, it cooperates in getting you back into shape with a vengeance—to the point where your body will surpass its previous fitness level. This holds true even when you are forced to take a layoff of weeks or even months. Athletes who have sustained injuries and who have had to take time off can confirm this truth.

TAKING TIME OFF FOR SICKNESS

What about sickness? Suppose, for example, you have the flu. Of course, you cannot work out if you have a fever. In fact, if you tried to work out in such a condition, you'd probably be too weak to handle even the lightest weights, and after a few minutes, you would feel dizzy and would probably have to stop.

On the other hand, you don't want to baby yourself and give in to the slightest sniffle. If you feel a cold coming on, instead of saying to yourself, "I'm going to be sick," and immediately giving in to it, try to ward it off. Instead think, "I'm not going to let this cold invade my body." Then "tell" your immune system to fight off the invading germs. Picture your immune cells destroying the germ cells. Then work out as usual. You'll find that many times you can ward off what might otherwise have been a few-days layup if you use your mind as your ally.

WHAT ABOUT INJURY?

If you have sustained an injury, chances are you can work around it. For example, if you have broken your ankle, there's no reason why you can't exercise your upper body. If you've sprained your right arm, and it is in a cast, there's no reason why you can't try to perform your exercises with the cast on your arm, but carefully— and with lighter weights. I did this with a cast, and in fact, to my doctor's dismay, I wore off two casts. Of course, I'm not telling you to ignore your doctor's orders. After seeing how determined I was, my doctor reluctantly gave me his permission to work out, with the warning: "Be careful. Don't overdo it."

Many times doctors will actually recommend that you do exercise for an injured area. For example, those people who sustain knee injuries are often asked to do leg extensions as part of their healing therapy. The bottom line is, if you've sustained an injury, don't assume that now everything stops. You'd be surprised about how much you can do, even if you end up working with three-pound dumbbells and using dynamic tension, as described in *The 12-Minute Total-Body Workout*, as well as in Chapter 8, a system recommended by many doctors and chiropractors for those who are unable to do a full-weight workout due to injury.

It is always better to do something than to do nothing, not only for the body, but for the mind as well. Working around an injury tells you that you are still in control, and that all is not lost. It gives you the feeling that you are participating in your healing, rather than sitting around like a helpless victim.

WHAT IF YOU STOP WORKING OUT—WILL THE MUSCLES TURN TO FAT?

People often ask me this question because they are not sure they will want to keep this up forever, and they fear that if they don't keep it up, they will look worse than they did had they never worked out in the first place. They've been warned by people who have no knowledge of the psysiology of the human body that "if you stop working out, it will all turn to fat."

You can put your worries aside. Muscle cells and fat cells are completely different from each other—both structurally and functionally. It is physically impossible for muscle to turn to fat. What happens if you stop working out is your muscles eventually shrink back to the size they were before you started working out—and it takes about the same amount of time you worked out for this to happen.

For example, if you worked out for one year, and then stopped, it would take a year for your muscles to return to their original size. They would not be smaller than they were originally, nor would they be covered with fat. They would simply be what they were before. But there's good news if you ever want to start working out again.

The other aspect, the eventual shrinkage of muscle and, with it, the return of the metabolism to its slower rate, is the second cause of weight gain. But don't misunderstand. The metabolism does not slow down to a slower rate than it was originally—but rather to exactly what it used to be before you started working out. So there is absolutely nothing to lose and everything to gain by working out.

At best, you will work out forever and be healthy and happy, and at worst, you will stop working out and eventually be back to square one—but with a bonus: if you ever started working out again, you would get in shape in a third the time it took you before!

MUSCLE-BUILDING ENZYMES, CARBO PACKS, FAT BURNERS—DO THEY WORK?

As you go along in your workout, you will meet people who will suggest food supplements such as amino acid compounds to build muscle, carbo packs or drinks for increased energy, or special enzymes that claim to increase body heat in order to burn more fat. There is no proof whatsoever that any of these products work. Your best bet is to stay away from them. The most intelligent thing to do is to depend upon vitamin- and mineral-packed natural foods, such as the ones suggested in Chapter 9, and to continue to do the workout.

It is human nature to want to take short-cuts—but unfortunately, when it comes to the body, there is no other way to get and stay in shape but to follow the natural course of development—through healthful eating and consistent, appropriate exercise.

WHAT ABOUT LAGGING BODY PARTS?

If after three to six months, you notice that your chest, shoulders, biceps, triceps, or back (or calves or thighs, for those of you who have chosen to do the optional leg workout) are lagging behind, you can take advantage of the methods described on pp. 62–64. If, on the other hand, it is your abdominal area that is lagging behind, you don't have to wait three to six months. You can take action after three weeks.

Begin a "bombs away" program on your midsection. This program is found in *Gut Busters*, a stomach routine that offers seven exercises not found in this workout. Do the Gut Busters routine on every day that you do not exercise abdominals with the Top Shape Workout—except that you should take one day off a week. In other words, if you are on the three-day plan for Top Shape, and you work your stomach on Monday, Wednesday, and Friday, add Gut Busters on Tuesday, Thursday, and Saturday, and take Sunday off. If you are on a split routine, and you work your stomach on Monday, Tuesday, Thursday, and Saturday, do Gut Busters on Wednesday and Friday, and take Sunday off.

The idea is to bomb away at your abdominals six days a week, hitting them with exercises that challenge them from every conceivable angle. This will greatly speed up your progress and eventually give you the midsection that you see on champion bodybuilders (you will get "the boxes," sometimes called "beer cans").

HOW TO AVOID WORKOUT BOREDOM

You don't have to stick to the Top Shape Workout year-in and year-out. You can switch to my other programs, Bottoms Up, the Fat-Burning Workout, the 12-Minute Total-Body Workout, or Now or Never. What? Am I telling you to do a woman's workout? Of course not. The exercises in those books are exactly the same as those I prescribe for men (and by the way, women can do the Top Shape Workout too!), with the exception of the hip/buttocks exercises—which you will leave out, because unlike women, men do not have "childrearing hips." If a man wants to tighten his buttocks, he can do the thigh routine. It offers just the right amount of challenge to the gluteus maximus muscles.

The only other thing that is different about my books addressed to women is the "talk." When I'm talking to women, I naturally emphasize certain issues over other issues. So if you get one of my books addressed to women, and you come across an issue that does not involve men, just skip over it. But most of the information in those books will apply to men as well as women.

For those of you who want to take advantage of the giant set speed workout discussed in this book, I strongly suggest that you get a copy of *The Fat-Burning Workout*, because it clearly explains that system, and *is* in fact a complete giant set workout. There are up to five exercises per body part for each giant set, and there are also some exercises not presented in *Top Shape*, so you can use them for a change of pace.

The Fat-Burning Workout (and any giant set routine for that matter) will help you to burn maximum fat, while at the same time give your muscles maximum definition. It's a good idea to switch to this workout for a few months each year, just before the summer, so that your body will appear lean and defined for the beach season. This giant set system is, in fact, exactly what champion bodybuilders use right before contests, when they are not looking to add on much size, but are rather interested in burning off that last bit of fat and achieving maximum hardness and definition for contest day.

Another change of pace can be the 12-Minute Total-Body Workout. If you are feeling burned out from working out, and would like to do less, but you don't want to stop working out completely (something you should never do), you can switch to this routine for a few weeks, or even for a few months. Then, when you go back to a regular workout, such as Top Shape, the Fat-Burning Workout or Now or Never, you'll find that you have not lost muscle tone—and, in addition, that you do not experience inordinate soreness the day after working out—because your muscles will have been kept challenged.

Finally, if you want a workout that is very similar to Top Shape, but would like some different exercises, try Now or Never for a while. That book also has information that is not found in any of my other books.

But don't try anything new until you have used this program for six months—even a year. It's better to get used to one routine and to have it down pat, before switching around. How much switching should you do? Let your body be your guide. As long as you are working out—doing one of the routines, you won't get out of shape. Your body will tell you which routine is best for its needs—but once again, don't try this until you have gotten into shape and stayed there for a few months (six months to a year), so that your body will know what it's doing. If you try it too soon, your body will become confused.

FOR A REAL TREAT, TAKE A FITNESS VACATION

When going on vacation to relax, most people think in terms of going to an island and lying in the sun or the shade with a cool drink—and just vegetating. But there's another way to go. You can try a fitness vacation for a change of pace. There are literally hundreds of health spas all over the country, where you can go to relax, and at the same time give your body and mind a real treat.

One of my favorite places to go is Canyon Ranch. They have two facilities, one in Tucson, Arizona, and one in the Berkshires in Massachusetts. They offer a delicious menu of low-fat foods, outdoor activities such as walks, hikes, canoe rides, and bike rides, and they have all sorts of indoor exercise activities—up to and including a fully equipped gym with a generous supply of free weights and all of the latest machines. They also have inspirational guest speakers (I dare say, I have been one of them) and fitness consultants that will sit down with you and map out a program especially designed for your needs. In addition, and sometimes I feel that this is the best part, they offer massages and treatments, of every kind.

Canyon Ranch is not the only facility that offers such services. Take a look at *The Ultimate Spa Book* (see bibliography), which gives details on hundreds of spas, so that you can determine which spa is best suited to your needs and to your budget.

If your health is your primary concern, the Pritikin Longevity Center (either in Miami or Santa Monica) is the place for you. Men and women of all ages come to the centers—some who have heart disease, diabetes, high blood pressure, blood cholesterol problems, gout, and claudication. Others come in order to prevent future health problems. The centers have one goal: helping the guest to get healthy and stay healthy for the rest of his or her life.

First, your health will be fully evaluated by a staff doctor, who will then oversee your progress and personally supervise your diet and exercise program. During your stay, you will learn completely new eating and cooking habits. In addition, you will be able to keep up your Top Shape Workout, because now the Pritikin Institute has a special room with benches and dumbbells.

THEY WOULD RATHER FIGHT THAN QUIT!

A final word of encouragement is in order. I asked several men who got into shape with this program if they would ever give it up. Each of them quickly replied that they would never think of such a thing. Then I said, "What about if I offered you money—how much would it take for you to promise to give up this program?" "It would be big bucks," said one man. "I mean, a brand-new Jaguar ... no, no. I wouldn't do it for that, even for any money. I couldn't put a price on it. No deal."

"You can't count it in money," said another man. "You're not talking about just looks. You're talking about my health and my job. Who knows, if I let myself go, I might lose my job—you can't put a price on that these days—especially in the white-collar field. And never mind that. For the first time in many years, I feel alive and young. No. You can't pay me enough to stop."

"If you don't have physical fitness, you have nothing, so how can you talk about a price," says a third man. "It isn't even a question to be considered. In fact, after a month, I knew that this would be something I would do for life. Now, for sure, I'm past the point of no return. I wouldn't give it up no matter what you offered me."

I'd love to hear from *you*. Please write to me at my P.O. Box, and let me know how you feel about the workout. Also, feel free to ask questions. I will personally answer every letter, *if you include a stamped, self-addressed envelope.* Also, if you wish to order dumbbells, an exercise bench, or any other item, please write to me at the following P.O. Box:

Joyce L. Vedral
P.O. Box 7433
Wantagh, NY 11793

Cast-Iron Dumbbells
Set of 5-pound dumbbells, $17.98
Set of 8-pound dumbbells, $24.98
Set of 10-pound dumbbells, $29.98
Set of 12-pound dumbbells, $34.98
Set of 15-pound dumbbells, $39.98
Set of 20-pound dumbbells, $43.98
Set of 25-pound dumbbells, $47.98
Set of 30-pound dumbbells, $51.99
Set of 35-pound dumbbells, $55.00
Set of 40-pound dumbbells, $59.00

Add 50 cents per pound for shipping and handling. In doing your calculations, remember to double the weight of the dumbbells, since there are two dumbbells in each set. In other words, if you order a set of 10-pound dumbbells, the total shipping weight is 20 pounds. At 50 cents a pound, your total shipping weight will be $10.00. (Note that dumbbells are expensive to ship. If you have a gym supply store nearby, you will save a lot of money by purchasing them there. However, if it is inconvenient for you to get to the store, you may feel that it's worth the price to take advantage of this service.)

Personalized Flat-Incline-Decline Exercise Bench
(As seen in the photographs in Chapter 6.)
$159.98 plus $19.02 shipping and handling; total: $179.00
The bench is made of white steel with black, thickly padded upholstery, with my signature.

Leather Ball Bearing Jump Rope
8 ft (for people 5' 11" and under) $21.98 plus $3.00 shipping; total: $24.98
9½ ft (for people 6' and over) $24.98 plus $3.00 shipping; total: $27.98

BMI Stepper with Multi-Function Electronic Monitor
$149.98 plus $19.02 shipping and handling; total: $169.00

Healthtrainer by Maximus Fitness
(As seen in photographs in Chapter 7.)
$998.99 plus $99.01 shipping; total: $1,098.00
To order the Healthtrainer or request more information about this item before
purchasing, write to:

> Lud Shusterich
> 3475 Old Conejo Road
> Newbury Park, CA 91320
> or call 805 498-0455

All items are shipped UPS.

Bibliography

OTHER FITNESS BOOKS AUTHORED AND CO-AUTHORED BY JOYCE VEDRAL

Vedral, Joyce, Ph.D. *Bottoms Up!* New York: Warner Books, 1993.

Vedral, Joyce, Ph.D. *Gut Busters.* New York: Warner Books, 1992.

Vedral, Joyce, Ph.D. *The Fat-Burning Workout.* Warner Books, 1991. (The two-volume video of this book is available in all stores, or see ordering information below)

Vedral, Joyce, Ph.D. *The 12-Minute Total-Body Workout.* New York: Warner Books, 1989.

Vedral, Joyce, Ph.D. *Now or Never.* New York: Warner Books, 1986.

Vedral, Marthe, and Joyce Vedral, Ph.D. *The College Dorm Workout.* New York: Warner Books, 1994.

Weider, Betty, and Joyce L. Vedral, Ph.D. *Better and Better.* New York: Dell Publishing Company, 1993.

Kneuer, Cameo, and Joyce L. Vedral, Ph.D. *Cameo Fitness.* New York: Warner Books, 1990.

Portuguese, Gladys, and Joyce L. Vedral, Ph.D. *The Hard Bodies Express Workout.* New York: Dell Publishing Company, 1988.

McLish, Rachel, and Joyce L. Vedral, Ph.D. *Perfect Parts.* New York: Warner Books, 1987.

Portuguese, Gladys, and Joyce L. Vedral, Ph.D. *Hard Bodies.* Dell Publishing Company, 1986

VIDEO

Bottoms Up!, by Joyce L. Vedral, Good Times Video. Volume I: "Upper Body Workout"; Volume II: "Lower Body Workout"; Volume III: "Middle Body Workout." Each volume is $19.98 and available at local video stores, or call 1-800-433-6769.

Most of the exercises in Chapter 6 are illustrated in these videos.

NUTRITION, DIET, SPAS, AND COOKBOOKS

Donkersloot, Mary, R.D. *The Fast-Food Diet: Quick and Healthy Eating at Home and On the Go.* New York: Simon & Shuster, 1991. (Use the charts in the book to stay within my fat gram recommendation of thirty to forty grams per day. Fat grams are listed for meals from Italian, Chinese, Mexican, as well as fast-food restaurants. You'll even find snacks, desserts, cereals, and frozen foods.)

Katahan, Martin, Ph.D. and Jamie Pope-Curdle, M.S., R.D. *The T-Factor Fat Gram Counter.* New York: W.W. Norton & Company, 1989.

Kirshbaum, John (ed). *The Nutrition Almanac.* New York: McGraw-Hill, 1989.

Mycoskie, Pam. *Butter Busters*™, New York: Warner Books, 1994.

Natow, Annette B., Ph.D., R.D., and Jo-Ann Heslin, M.A., R.D. *The Fat Attack Plan.* New York: Pocket Books, 1990.

Reynolds, Bill, and Joyce Vedral, Ph.D. *Supercut: Nutrition for the Ultimate Physique.* Chicago: Contemporary Books, 1987.

Sarnoff, Pam Martin. *The Ultimate Spa Book.* New York: Warner Books, 1989.

Spear, Ruth. *Low Fat and Loving It: How to Lower Your Fat Intake and Still Eat the Foods You Love—200 Recipes.* New York: Warner Books, 1991.

MAGAZINES AND NEWSLETTERS FOR EXERCISE AND NUTRITION INFORMATION

American Health, 80 Fifth Avenue, New York, NY 10011.
Longevity, 1965 Broadway, New York, NY 10023-5965.
Men's Fitness, 21100 Erwin Street, Woodand Hills, CA 91367.
Muscle and Fitness, 21100 Erwin Street, Woodand Hills, CA 91367.
Your Health, 540 N.W. Broken Sound Boulevard, Boca Raton, FL 33431.
Mayo Clinic Nutrition Letter, 200 First Street, S.W., Rochester, MN 55905.
Tufts University Diet and Nutrition Letter, P.O. Box 57857, Boulder, CO 80322-7857.
University of California, Berkeley, Wellness Letter, Health Letter Associates. P.O. Box 420148, Palm Coast, FL 32142.

SELF-HELP BOOKS AUTHORED BY JOYCE VEDRAL

For Parents

My Teenager Is Driving Me Crazy. New York: Ballantine Books, 1989.
How to Get Your Kids to Talk. New York: Ballantine Books, 1993.

For Teens

I Dare You. New York: Ballantine Books, 1983.
My Parents Are Driving Me Crazy. New York: Ballantine Books, 1986.
I Can't Take It Anymore. New York: Ballantine Books, 1987.
The Opposite Sex Is Driving Me Crazy. New York: Ballantine Books, 1988.
Boyfriends: Getting Them, Keeping Them, Living Without Them. New York: Ballantine Books, 1990.
My Teacher Is Driving Me Crazy. New York: Ballantine Books, 1991.

For Women and Men Who Want to Learn How Women Think

Get Rid of Him. New York: Warner Books, 1993.

The parent books and all of the teen books can be ordered by calling 1-800-733-3000. The other Vedral books can be found in or ordered from your local bookstore.

Index

F

G

H

I

J

K

L

Y

About the Author

Joyce Vedral, a Ph.D. in English literature (New York University) got her start in fitness writing at *Muscle and Fitness* and *Men's Fitness* magazines, where she regularly interviewed champion bodybuilders—learning their secrets and interpreting them for "the average Joe," as she puts it.

In time, Joyce noticed a lack of weight-training workout books for people who are *not* interested in looking like "Arnold," but who would like to be in great shape—without spending hours a day. Joyce began writing workout books for the average person in 1986 and since then has influenced almost two million men and women—who would now rather "fight than quit" using one of her workouts. The reason books like *Gut Busters, Bottoms Up!, The Fat-Burning Workout, Now or Never, The 12-Minute Total-Body Workout,* and *The College Dorm Workout* have sold so well is simple: they achieve the promised results.

But there's another reason for Joyce's success: Joyce, with her trademark upbeat voice, is a real person who convinces people in lectures and on television shows all over the country that "if I can do it, if my Uncle Dave can do it, if the before-and-after men and women in the book can do it, so can you."

Joyce is a frequent guest on *Oprah Winfrey, Geraldo, Donahue, Sally Jessy Raphael, Montel Williams, Joan Rivers,* and CNN's *Sonya Live,* and has been written up in the *New York Times,* the *Daily News,* and the *New York Post.* She is a sought-after speaker for corporate groups, fitness centers, and shopping malls across the country.